Renata Faria

Interface between abutment and implant

Renata Faria

Interface between abutment and implant

Evaluation of bacterial infiltration

ScienciaScripts

Imprint

Any brand names and product names mentioned in this book are subject to trademark, brand or patent protection and are trademarks or registered trademarks of their respective holders. The use of brand names, product names, common names, trade names, product descriptions etc. even without a particular marking in this work is in no way to be construed to mean that such names may be regarded as unrestricted in respect of trademark and brand protection legislation and could thus be used by anyone.

Cover image: www.ingimage.com

This book is a translation from the original published under ISBN 978-613-9-64161-1.

Publisher:
Sciencia Scripts
is a trademark of
Dodo Books Indian Ocean Ltd. and OmniScriptum S.R.L publishing group

120 High Road, East Finchley, London, N2 9ED, United Kingdom
Str. Armeneasca 28/1, office 1, Chisinau MD-2012, Republic of Moldova, Europe
Printed at: see last page
ISBN: 978-620-7-76278-1

DEDICATORY

To my husband Wagner, my companion in both happy and difficult times, for all his love and affection, support and encouragement. Thank you for encouraging me to realise my ideals.

To my sons Vitor and Heitor, my passions. To you I dedicate this work and all my love.

To my parents Sylvio and Lored, examples of dignity and dedication to their children, for all their love, affection and care in my personal and professional development. Without you, the difficulties might not have been overcome. Thank you very much.

To my siblings Valéria, Silvana, Marcos Fábio and Marcos Flávio, who make our house a real home.

To my in-laws Dario and Mariângela, who took me in as their daughter. You have my respect and admiration.

SPECIAL THANKS

To my supervisor, Professor Marco Antonio Bottino, whose example of dedication and professional success inspires our deepest admiration, thank you very much for the opportunity and for showing me different paths and new horizons. My special love to the master and friend.

To Mariângela Duarte, for her valuable collaboration in acquiring the necessary and fundamental equipment for the development of our research, and for her incessant struggle for the improvement of education in our country.

To my dear and wise friend Fernanda Pelógia Camargo, a postgraduate colleague who was always there and willing to help.

To Silvia H. Barbosa, a special friend, cheerful, intelligent and dedicated. I can't thank you enough for all you've helped. It's great to be around people like you.

To my friend Liliana Gressler May, always cheerful and patient. Thank you for your partnership throughout this period, helping and working alongside me.

To Daniele Paschoto, for her invaluable collaboration in this work.

To Diana, a friend of many years. Thank you for your valuable help.

ACKNOWLEDGEMENTS

To my doctoral colleagues, Fernanda, Graziela, Renata, Alfredo and Nori, for their harmonious and pleasant coexistence.

To my fellow postgraduate students, Aleska, Aline, Anderson, Celina, Eurípedes, Guilherme, Humberto, Liliana, Lucas, Luis Gustavo, Mariana, Priscila, Regina, Rodrigo, Sandra, Sheila, Silvia M., and Susana.

To my colleague Luciane Dias de Oliveira, for her collaboration in preparing the samples and the apparatus for our methodology, who was always available and patient.

To Universidade Estadual Paulista "Julio de Mesquita Filho", in the person of the Director of the Sào José dos Campos School of Dentistry, Prof. Dr. José Roberto Rodrigues; to the Department of Dental Materials and Prosthodontics, and to the Postgraduate Programme in Restorative Dentistry - Prosthodontics, for the opportunity to complete my doctorate.

To the professors of the Postgraduate Programme in Restorative Dentistry - Prosthodontics, for their teaching and pleasant interaction.

To the Department of Bioscience and Oral Diagnosis for the opportunity to discover new paths in research.

To Prof Antonio Olavo Cardoso Jorge, for his help with the methodology of this work.

To the secretaries of the Postgraduate Programme, Erena, Lílian, Maria Aparecida and Rosemary, for their attention.

To Prof Ivan Balducci, for carrying out the statistical analysis of this work.

To Conexão Sistemas de Prótese, especially its directors Dr Rodolfo Candia Alba Jr. and Douglas Cândido Figueira, for the technical support and material made available for the research.

SUMMARY

SUMMARY

The aim of this study was to assess bacterial infiltration *in vitro at* the interface between the abutment and the implant, comparing three types of prosthetic connections: External Hexagon (HE), Indexed Internal Hexagon (HII) and Cone Morse (CM). Under sterile conditions, an *Escherichia coli colony* was inoculated into the apical portion of the abutment screw. The abutments were then fixed to the implants with a torque of 20 N/cm. Samples with immediate external contamination were discarded. The samples were placed in test tubes containing 2 ml of sterile TSB broth. After daily monitoring for 7 days, the broths that were turbid were seeded in petri dishes with TSA and incubated in a bacteriological oven at 37°C for 24 hours to observe bacterial growth. Gram staining was carried out on both the broth and the colony resulting from the sowing to check for the presence of *E. coli* (Gram-negative). At the end of the period, all the samples were separated, the internal contents were collected with a paper cone and saline solution and sown in petri dishes containing TSA, taken to a bacteriological oven at 37ᵉ C for 24 hours to check the viability of the bacteria. Samples that did not contain viable *E.coli* were discarded from the final result. After discarding the samples due to external contamination and viability, the following sample numbers were obtained: 38 (HE), 40 (HII) and 41 (CM). The results, in % of samples with bacterial infiltration, were subjected to the multiple comparisons of proportions test. Survival curves were analysed using the Kaplan-Meyer method and compared using the Log-Rank statistical test. There was no difference between HE (10.53%), HII (4.88%) and CM (7.50%). The survival curves did not differ. Bacterial infiltration occurred similarly in the three types of connections between abutments and implants, despite the different interface configurations.

Keywords: Dental implants; prostheses and implants; microbiology; biomechanics.

CHAPTER 1

INTRODUCTION

Brânemark[9] , in 1983, observed osseointegration when titanium implants were inserted into medullary cavities and, after a period of healing, a layer of compact bone was found around the implants without any interposition of soft tissue. After different studies, he defined osseointegration as a direct structural and functional connection between living bone and the surface of a load-bearing implant. The basic concepts of osseointegration evolved from various experimental and clinical studies carried out in Sweden since 1952, aimed at studying the reaction of bone marrow to various traumas and clinical procedures[10] . At the beginning of the 1960s, these studies revealed the possibility of establishing real osseointegration of titanium with bone tissue. Thus, the first edentulous patient was treated with titanium implants in 1965[2] , according to the principles of osseointegration. The high levels of success reported by these Swedish researchers[11] are now being achieved by dentists all over the world. The successful replacement of a lost natural tooth with an implant is one of the greatest clinical advances in dentistry[10,11] .

Longitudinal studies have shown that implants remain in function for a long time, where a conventional criterion for success is a bone loss of 1.5 mm during the first year of function after the installation of the prosthesis, and less than 0.2 mm every year[1,4,20,31,34] . This criterion is related to consistent observations of bone loss around external hexagon implants with their respective prophetic connections with the interface between abutments and implants located at the level of the bone Christian[11] . This phenomenon has also been confirmed in other studies[12,30] . However, although the implant remains in function, the possible sequelae of bone loss can negatively affect the aesthetic objectives. Peri-implant bone loss can lead to proportional gingival recession[12,28] , as occurs in the natural dentition, as demonstrated in a study of patients who had a lower papilla height due to the increased distance between the contact point of the teeth and the Christian bone .[48]

The literature identifies six categories of complications associated with prostheses on implants: surgical complications, implant loss, bone loss, peri-implant tissue complications, mechanical and aesthetic complications. Many studies have investigated the relationship between bone loss and implant loss and the factors commonly used to assess the periodontal condition of natural teeth (presence of plaque, oral hygiene, gingivitis, probing depth, bleeding on probing, microbiota present, distance from the prosthesis and soft tissues, and others). Zarb and Schmit[54] , 1993, reported that successful osseointegration can be maintained regardless of the patient's oral hygiene performance.

For Weber *et al.*[52] , 2000, there are few levels of correlation between clinical periodontal parameters and radiographic measurements of bone loss. According to the authors, these parameters are limited for determining a prognosis of future bone loss around implants. In contrast to these studies, many others report the existence of a relationship between factors used in the periodontal assessment of natural teeth and the success of implants. Mombelli and Lang[33] , 1994, associated implant failure with a high proportion of microorganisms related to periodontal disease. Henry *et al.*[27] ,1993 found that implant failures were more concentrated in patients with greater plaque accumulation. In the study by Block and Kent[8] ,1994, it was observed that lack of keratinisation of the gums and poor hygiene were some of the most common reasons for implant loss.

Inflammatory reactions around implants have not yet been adequately studied. These inflammations can influence the peri-implant gingival level, jeopardising aesthetics as well as tissue health. Using the conventional technique, the implant is installed at the level of the bone Christian and, after 3 to 6 months, a prosthetic abutment is installed to make the prosthesis, thus creating an interface (microfissure) between the abutment and the implant at the level of the bone Christian.

Broggini *et al.*[2] ,2003, have shown by evidence histomorphometrically, an infiltrate of inflammatory cells develops around the implants and can vary according to their design. In their study, an intense infiltrate of inflammatory cells (predominantly neutrophils) and significant bone loss were associated with the presence of microcracks in the Christian bone. Based on their histological study of lost implants, Covani *et al.*[44] , 2006, stated that the high bacterial colonisation observed at the interface between abutments and implants may legitimise the hypothesis that the microcrack formed at this interface presents a risk of bone loss.

The design of various implant systems requires 2 surgical stages, i.e. installation of the implant in the first stage and the prosthetic abutment in the second. However, as soon as the abutment is positioned on the implant, a gap is created at this interface, which is usually located at the level of or slightly below the bone Christian, making the region susceptible to microbial colonisation[28,30,44] . These spaces can act as niches for bacteria, leading to a loss of the peri-implant mucosal seal and changes in the clinical and microbiological parameters of the tissues. In this way, they can promote the development of pathologies and jeopardise the maintenance of osseointegration[1,12,28,30,31,35,37,51] . The presence of an infiltrate of inflammatory cells at the junction between the abutment and the implant, even with meticulous plaque control and clinically healthy soft tissue, has been shown in clinical research .[13,51]

The importance of the location of the crack formed at the interface between the abutment and the implant has been discussed in the literature. Studies have shown bone loss of more than 2mm with the interface at the level of the Christian bone[28,30]. Minimal bone loss was observed when non-submerged, 1-stage, gapless implant systems were used[28,30,37]. In contrast, in a histomorphometric study, no difference was observed in the dimensions of the peri-implant mucosa, junctional epithelium, connective tissue and bone loss for interfaces positioned at different depths in the bone.[49]

Attempts have been made to achieve a more rigid connection between the abutment and the implant. Basically, external prosthetic connections of the external hexagon type and internal connections such as: hexagonal, conical (cone morse) or a combination of both are used in implant rehabilitations. Conical connections seem to have superior stability compared to external hexagon connections[32,53]. According to Dibart *et* al.[17], 2005, the friction connection of a conical abutment is a cold weld, metal to metal, creating a seal, making the interface between the abutment and the implant too narrow for bacteria to pass through.

Research *in* iz/tro [3,5,15,16,17,19,23,26,29,36,46,47,50] e *in* v/vo[13,38,42,45], has evaluated bacterial infiltration of the interfaces between abutments and implants with various types of prosthetic configurations. The results are highly controversial.

From a technical point of view, gaps between components are inevitable when adapting the different parts of the abutment and implant assembly, but their clinical significance has been neglected by manufacturers and clinicians. We believe that the occurrence of bacterial infiltration is one of the parameters used to analyse the quality of these connections, which currently come in various configurations. The aim of this study was therefore to evaluate the behaviour of different types of prosthetic connections in relation to bacterial infiltration through the interfaces between abutments and implants.

CHAPTER 2

LITERATURE REVIEW

Considering the various aspects addressed in this study, we decided to divide the literature review into four items: 1 - Rehabilitation with implants; 2 - Mechanical aspects of prosthetic connections for implants; 3 - Biological aspects of connections between prosthetic abutments and implants; 4 - Infiltration at the interface between abutment and implant.

2.1 Rehabilitation with implants

Brânemark[9] , in 1983, reviewed the studies and advances in osseointegration. According to the author, osseointegration was observed when titanium implants were introduced into medullary cavities, and followed by an adequate healing period, a layer of compact cortical bone was found around the implants without any apparent soft tissue intervention between the normal bone and the implant surface. The author observed a direct correlation between the titanium surface, the absence of contamination, the healing period and the histological pattern of the adjacent bone. According to the author, the anchoring capacity of an implant in the mandible is 100kg and 30 to 50kg in the maxilla. Osseointegration begins with the placement of the implant, which must be immobilised in the bone tissue immediately after installation. After a period of healing, vital bone tissue is in close contact with the surface of the fixture, without any other intermediate tissue. The osseointegrated implant is directly connected to bone tissue capable of undergoing remodelling according to the direction and magnitude of the masticatory loads applied. Osseointegration can be compromised when there is excessive trauma during surgery, infection or excessive loading during the healing phase. In these cases, the formation of connective tissue replaces the development of bone tissue, jeopardising implant anchorage. The author states that there is a correlation between the titanium implant and adjacent hard and soft tissues, which eventually improves anchorage over the years.

Henry *et aF*[7] in 1993 carried out a retrospective study of fifty-nine patients with Branemark implants. The clinical parameters assessed were biofilm indices, gingivitis, sulcus depth, bleeding after probing, mobility, prosthesis stability and stomatognathic function, and the bone level assessed radiographically. After three years, 460 implants supporting 174 prostheses in 139 patients were evaluated. The results suggest that treatment success in partially edentulous patients is comparable to that of fully edentulous patients.

In 1993, Zarb and Schimitt[54] evaluated the clinical results of edentulous patients treated with osseointegrated implants. Forty-six patients wearing full dentures were selected for the study, forty of whom required mandibular treatment, three maxillary treatment and three in both arches. Four to six implants were placed using the submerged technique. The implants were placed between the mental foramen in the mandible and between the first premolars in the maxilla. After six months of healing, the prophetic abutments were connected and 46 implant-supported fixed partial dentures and three overdentures were made. All patients were satisfied with the treatment. Eighty-nine per cent of the implants remained osseointegrated after nine years. The records were divided into three groups: A) all implants placed in the 35 arches were osseointegrated. Fixed partial dentures were made for 32 arches and overdentures for three arches. Twenty-one implants failed to osseointegrate and were removed during the second surgical stage. B) failures occurred in 10 arches (one in each) and as four or more implants remained integrated, treatment proceeded as planned. C) four patients formed this group, with inadequate or insufficient support that excluded the possibility of using implant-supported prostheses. After nine years of treatment with osseointegrated implants, implant-supported fixed partial dentures and overdentures were considered a clinical success.

In 1994, Block and Kent[8] evaluated hydroxyapatite-covered implants placed between 1985 and 1988 and between 1989 and 1991 in relation to factors associated with success or failure. The implants were followed up for 4 to 8 years or 1 to 4 years, depending on the period in which they were placed. Success or failure ratios, time to failure, outcome after implant removal and morbidity analysis were evaluated. After seven to eight years, the success rate was 86.5 per cent when the mandible and maxilla were considered, 84.2 per cent for maxillary implants and 87.5 per cent for mandibular implants. For implants evaluated between one and four years, the success rate was 97.5%, 97.5% for maxillary implants and 97.6% for mandibular implants. The difference between the periods was statistically significant for the maxilla in the anterior region. A regression analysis indicates that failures did not follow a linear progression in relation to time. The most common reasons for failure were lack of keratinised gingiva, poor oral hygiene, excessive occlusal forces and malposition. Comparison with other implant systems revealed that the success rate was comparable to that of other implant systems.

Ekfeldt eial.[20] , in 1994, carried out a retrospective study of patients with single prostheses on Brânèmark implants after a short period of time. They assessed 77 patients who had 94 two-stage implants placed between 1987 and 1990. One implant placed in the anterior maxilla failed when the prosthetic abutment was connected. The observation time ranged from 14 to 55 months and the restorations were in function from three to 46 months. Factors such as gingiva, plaque, calculus, implant stability and aesthetics were analysed. Radiographs were taken to assess osseointegration and bone loss. A questionnaire was given to each patient. One implant failed during the first year in function. Fifty-eight per cent of the prostheses were screw-retained and 42% cement-retained. Gingivitis was found in 26 per cent and visible plaque in 13 per cent. No calculus was found around any of the implants. Two fistulas were found associated with prosthetic abutments with mobility. The predominant complication was screw loss (40%). The aesthetic evaluation was similar between evaluators and patients: 46% considered the treatment very good, 37% good, 17% acceptable. In radiographic examinations, bone loss was found in 14 implants, ranging from 0.6 to 1.8 mm. Loss of osseointegration was found in one implant.

In 1996, Avivi-Arber and Zarb[4] evaluated the results of implant-supported prostheses using osseointegration analysis and success criteria. Forty-one patients were selected with single-unit prosthetic spaces for implant-supported prostheses according to the two-stage technique. Forty-nine Brânèmark implants were placed in different regions of the jaws (30 in the upper incisor and canine regions, 5 in the upper premolar and molar regions, 1 in the lower incisor and canine region and 1 in the lower molar region). The length of the implants varied between 10 and 20 mm and the diameter between 3.75 and 4 mm. The healing period after the first surgical stage was four to six months. Thirty-eight patients with 45 implants were followed up after the restorations had been loaded. Different systems were used to make the prosthetic part and the type of prosthetic abutment was chosen depending on the region. Patients were assessed at one, six and twelve months after prosthetic completion. At each assessment, the crowns were removed and each implant was assessed clinically and radiographically. At the last assessment, all implants were asymptomatic and immobile. No inflammation was observed in the adjacent teeth and the gingival tissue was healthy. Bone loss ranged from 0.36 to 0.4 mm in the first year and averaged 0.2 mm per year. Loss of the prosthetic abutment or screw was the most common clinical complication. Fracture of the porcelain cover occurred in four crowns. According to the authors, treatment with implant-supported prostheses showed satisfactory results and promising performance.

Esposito *et al.*[2] \ in 1998, carried out a literature review on the factors that contribute to osseointegrated implant failures. According to the authors, failures can be divided into biological and mechanical. Other failures can be classified as iatrogenic, due to poor implant positioning or insufficient patient adaptation. Biological failures are those in which the host is inadequate in establishing (primary failures) or maintaining osseointegration (late failures). The parameters currently used to consider success are: absence of mobility, bone Christian loss of less than 1.5 mm during the first year and less than 0.2 mm annually and absence of pain and paresthesia; in addition, some authors consider the periodontal aspects of sulcus depth and gingival bleeding. The clinical signs of infection during the healing period are: secretion, fistulas, suppuration, tissue dehiscence and osteomyelitis, pain and mobility and can increase the chance of implant osseointegration failure. Different types of mobility can be found: 1) rotation, 2) lateral or horizontal, 3) axial or vertical, as well as different degrees of mobility. Other signs should be analysed, such as radiographic signs, where a radiolucent image around the implants suggests a lack of bone contact with the implant, as well as percussion signs. Progressive loss of bone Christian height is a clear sign of future implant loss. An implant is considered lost when bone loss reaches the apical 1/3 of the implant. Radiographic examination, although difficult to reproduce during evaluations, is more reliable than periodontal probing. There is no correlation between bleeding and radiographic and histological changes. An increase in the peridontal pocket around implants is related to a high degree of inflammation of the periodontal tissue, but not necessarily bone loss. In relation to the survey carried out on implant success rates, the authors observed that fixed partial dentures work better than implant-supported complete dentures. Primary and total failures of single-unit prostheses show a low prevalence of fracture. An average failure rate of 7.3 per cent is considered acceptable, depending on the complexity and risks of the procedures. Implants placed after bone grafts have a higher failure rate of 14.9% after 2 years. Implants placed in the maxilla are less successful than those in the mandible, with the exception of partially edentulous patients, where performance is similar between the arches. The prevalence of failures due to peri-implantitis is extremely low (2.8 per cent). According to the authors, further studies should be conducted in order to establish the main causes of implant failure.

Esposito et al[22], in 1998, carried out a literature review on the factors associated with biological failures in the osseointegration of oral implants. The factors contributing to osseointegration failures were divided into endogenous (systemic and local) and exogenous (related to materials and the operator). Among the endogenous factors, the authors noted that age and genetic factors can alter bone mineral composition, collagen production, bone protein morphology and the bone's ability to heal. The patient's general health, such as nutritional status and general diseases such as metabolic, rheumatic, hormonal and immunological ones, can also affect osseointegration capacity. A consensus has also been established on the negative factors of smoking patients on implant survival. Among local factors, bone quality and quantity, as well as anatomical location, have a profound influence on the number of implant failures. In general, a large number of failures occur in the maxilla and in the posterior segment of both arches, which is partly explained by the different types of bone quality and loading conditions in these regions. With regard to bone grafts, a strong correlation has been observed between the complexity of the procedure during grafting and osseointegration failures. With regard to parafunction, it is generally agreed that excessive loads can induce bone loss. No correlation has been found between severe bouts of previous periodontitis and implant loss and, on the contrary, scientific evidence tends to reject this hypothesis, just as no correlation has been found between the amount of keratinised gingiva and implant failure. The indication for implant placement in patients who have undergone radiotherapy is delicate, as these patients have bone resorption, fibrosis and avascular necrosis. Among the exogenous factors, the operator factor has a major influence on the number of implant failures. Clinical experience reduces the number of failures. Ergonomics also has a major influence on the outcome of therapy. The heat generated during implant placement is associated with bone damage, which can jeopardise integration, as can the size of the microgap between implant and prosthetic abutment. Other factors are anchoring in bi-cortical bone and the placement of multiple implants, which can jeopardise the healing period. The presence of bacteria can interfere with the healing process if the host is unable to eliminate the pathogenic microorganisms, which generates an inflammatory process and leads to the loss of the implant. Exposure of the implant to immediate or premature loads is associated with an increase in implant failures. However, not only the quality but also the different characteristics of the implants have a major influence on the success of osseointegration. In fact, implants with a rough surface or apposition are associated with a low prevalence of failures.

Weber *et al.*[52] conducted a 5-year retrospective study in 2000 on the clinical longevity of implants and the correlation between changes in bone level and clinical success parameters. Clinical (suppuration, plaque, bleeding, sulcus depth, mobility and gingival condition) and radiographic examinations were carried out on 112 ITI implants inserted at different locations in the dental arches every year for 5 years. Ninety-nine per cent of the implants were considered a clinical success after 5 years. The average Christian bone loss was 0.6 mm in the first year and 0.05 mm annually. No statistically significant difference was found in bone loss during each year of assessment, suggesting that there was no bone loss during the osseointegration period. A low level of correlation was found between clinical signs and Christian bone loss, suggesting that clinical signs are limited in predicting bone loss.

In 2000, O'Mahony *et aP[5]* evaluated implants that had failed in order to identify characteristics that may have contributed to treatment failure. Forty-five implants that failed in patients without significant factors contributing to implant loss, such as smoking or diabetes, after an average of four years in function, were examined using SEM. The various types of implant placed showed areas of plaque retention along the prosthetic abutment/implant interface, the prosthetic abutment/prosthesis interface, on the surface of the abutment, the prosthesis and the implant. The size of the gap between the implant components, the surface roughness of the prostheses and abutments, the treated surface and the implant threads contributed to plaque accumulation and were favourable media for bacterial colonisation, which may be a primary factor in the development of peri-implant inflammation and the consequent loss of the implant.

Ricci *et al.[44]* conducted a retrospective study in 2004 on the clinical performance of implants subjected to masticatory loads for sixty months. Fifty-one patients were treated with 112 Frialit-2 implants using the submerged technique. Radiographs were taken every six months. After the implants had been loaded for five years, clinical and radiographic examinations were carried out. Plaque index, bleeding after probing and sulcus depth were the criteria measured during the clinical examination. The amount of bone Christian resorption was measured using radiographs. After five years, all the implants were intact. Seventy-one per cent of the implants had bone loss of less than 3 mm, 24% had between 3 and 5 mm and 4.5% had more than 5 mm. Bacterial plaque was not detected in 58 per cent, while 42 per cent had plaque in at least one region. Eighty-four per cent showed no gingival inflammation, while 15% had gingival bleeding. In seventy-one per cent, the probing did not exceed 3 mm, it was between 3 and 5 mm for 24% and greater than 5 mm for 4.5%. According to the authors, control can limit bone loss in two-stage implants.

2.2 Mechanical aspects of prophetic implant connections.

Binon[6] , in 1996, evaluated the influence of the mismatch between the hexagons of the implants and UCLA abutments on the stability of the fixation screws during function simulation. Ten groups of abutments were specially manufactured with modifications to the size of the hexagons, which were incrementally increased by 0.005 inches. They increased in size from 0.1065 to 0.1110 inches. The abutments were connected to the implants with a torque of 30Ncm. An off-axis load of 133 N was applied for 1150 cycles per minute and with 28 anti-clockwise rotations per minute to determine the stability of the abutment screw. The rotational misfit between the hexagons of the abutments and implants ranged from 1.94 degrees for abutments with smaller hexagons to 14.87 degrees for abutments with larger hexagons. The occurrence of screw loosening ranged from 134,000 to 9.3 million cycles. This study indicates that there is a direct correlation between hexagon maladaptation and screw loss from the prophetic abutment. The greater the rotational freedom, the greater the likelihood of abutment screw loosening.

Merz *et al.*[32] , in 2000, evaluated the behaviour of conical and conventional connections during mechanical cycling using finite element analysis. The model was created based on an ITI implant with a prosthetic abutment 6 degrees inclined and 7 mm high. The implants were immersed in polymethylmethacrylate resin and a 2 mm bone resorption was simulated. A circular-shaped alloy crown was represented, where the mechanical cycling load was applied. A non-linear contact was simulated between the prosthetic abutment and the conical connection. To demonstrate the effect associated with the eight-degree conical connection, an implant with an external hexagon connection was simulated. The first load simulation was clamping with 35 Nem of force. A calculation was carried out to determine the amount of force applied to

the prosthetic abutments were tightened and an additional load of 380 N was introduced at angles of 0, 15 and 30 degrees. The first load applied, for tightening, generated a symmetrical distribution of forces in both models. The conical connection resulted in wedge effects in the first 2 threads during cycling. Significantly higher levels of stress were generated in the external hexagon implant. At an angulation of 45[e] , the conical connection was able to absorb the stress generated, but the pre-stress in the threads increased. With the load applied at 15[S] , the tendency was to develop bending forces and compression areas. The majority of load transfer occurred in the conical connection, while in the external hexagon connection, tensile forces were observed in the threads and bending forces were distributed in the prophetic abutment portion. The results showed superior stability in the conical connections.

Weiss *et al.*[53] , in 2000, compared the loss of torque resistance after consecutive closures in different implant-prosthetic abutment systems. Seven systems were tested: 1) ITI Strauman - cone morse; 2) Alph Bio - cone morse; 3) Spline Calcitek - *Spline',* 4) Integral Calcitek - flat edge interface; 5) Steri-oss straight - external hexagon; 6)Omniloc Calcitek - internal octagon; 7) Brânemark Nobel - external hexagon. The torque was applied using a digital torque wrench by the same operator. For each abutment, the test was carried out as follows: the abutment was connected with a torque of 20Ncm, maintained for 5 seconds. After 10 seconds, the abutment was unscrewed and the removal torque measured. The abutment was then tightened again. The torque and removal cycles were repeated two hundred times. A progressive decrease in removal torque values was obtained in all systems. The removal torque loss values recorded were: 1) 0.5 Nem (ITI Strauman); 2) 0.6 Nem (Alph Bio); 3) 31.2 Nem (Spline Calcitek); 4) 2.6 Nem (Integral Calcitek); 5) 3.4 Nem (Steri-oss); 6)
6.5 Ncm (Omniloc Calcitek); 7) 6.2Ncm (Brànemark Nobel). They concluded that repeated insertion and removal of abutments can cause loss of torque retention, varying between implant systems.

Ding *et aL*™, in 2003, compared, radiographically and microscopically, two different internal connections (internal octagon and Morse cone with an eight-degree inclination) after repeated torque and counter-torque cycles and after fatigue, corresponding to implant deformation. Thirty-six implants with a diameter of 4.1 mm and a length of 10 mm were used. Twenty-four were synOcta implants, twelve with a solid prosthetic abutment and twelve were screw-retained implants with solid prosthetic abutments. The implants were embedded in acrylic resin and the abutments connected with a torque force of 35Ncm. After two minutes, the torque capable of unscrewing the prosthetic abutment was realised and recorded, and this process was repeated three times. For the bending test, 7.5 mm high crowns were made and cemented with temporary cement to the prosthetic abutments. A compressive force was applied to the incisal region until failure was recorded. Initially, the synOcta implant and Octa prosthetic abutment set showed lower resistance to torque, as well as resistance to bending.

Faria *et al*[2] \ in 2008, examined the effect of mechanical cycling fatigue on the removal torque values of prosthetic abutments for implants. Twenty implants with a double internal configuration (Morse cone or indexed internal hexagon) (Conexão Sistemas de Prostótese, Brazil) were used to test two types of prosthetic connections. The samples were divided into 2 groups (n=10): G1- implant and solid cone morse abutment; G2 - implant and indexed abutment. All the abutments were torqued to 20 Nem, as recommended by the manufacturer, using a digital torque wrench, and were subjected to 500,000 cycles. The value of the abutment removal torque was subsequently recorded. The results showed that group G1 (12.01 ±3.53 N/cm) was statistically different from G2 (3.05±1.62 N/cm) (p-value = 0.0002< 0.05). The authors concluded that the Morse cone connection had a higher removal torque value and could be considered more stable.

2.3 Biological aspects of connections between prophetic abutments and implants

In 1994, Mombelli and Lang[33] discussed the microbiological aspect of the tissues adjacent to dental implants. The authors observed that there is a clear distinction between microorganisms that participate in a stable microbiota and those that participate in peri-implantitis. Anaerobic Gram-negative bacteria are present in peri-implant pathologies. These organisms can also be found in periodontitis and orofacial infections. Spirochetes are indicative of an anaerobic environment and are not found in the physiological flora around implants. Antimicrobial treatment aims to reduce anaerobic bacteria, but the cause-effect relationship between specific pathogens and tissue destruction is still debatable. Numerous factors can influence the health of peri-implant tissues, particularly during the healing phase. Bacterial infection can occur as a second phenomenon if osseointegration does not occur or is lost for some non-microbial reason. Studies show that there are different forms of peri-implant disease, including specific infections or failures unrelated to pathogenic microorganisms.

Abrahamsson *et al.*\ in 1999, evaluated the formation of peri-implant tissues of 2-stage implants placed following the submerged and non-submerged technique. Dog premolars were extracted and after three months, Astra Tech implants were placed at the level of the Christian bone. After two weeks, radiographs were taken. After three months, reopening was carried out and prosthetic abutments 1.5 or 3 mm high, angled at 45^2 , were connected to the implants. At this point, new implants were placed, the prosthetic abutments immediately connected and new X-rays taken. After 3 and 6 months, the radiographs were repeated and the gingival and biofilm indices were measured. After 9 months, the animals were sacrificed and the mandibles removed. The mandible segments were dehydrated and embedded in methylmethacrylate. Sections were then obtained and immersed in toluidine blue. The biopsies were immersed in EDTA and the bone tissue decalcified. The biopsies were then dehydrated, sectioned and immersed in toluidine blue. Histological analysis included measurements of the peri-implant mucosa, junctional epithelium, the level of the bone Christian and the edge of the implant-prosthetic abutment interface. The morphometric analysis assessed the composition of the connective tissue. Bone analysis assessed bone contact on the implant and bone density. Clinical evaluation revealed minimal biofilm and inflammation-free tissue. In the implants that used the submerged technique (control group), the bone level decreased by an average of 0.23 mm after 3 months and 0.19 mm between 3 and 9 months. For implants placed using the non-submerged technique (experimental group), bone loss between 3 and 9 months was 0.30 mm. The length of the mucosa was 3.0 and 3.2 mm, the junctional epithelium was 2 and 1.9 mm long and fibroblasts were 13 and 12 per cent in the control and experimental groups, respectively. The percentage of bone in contact with the implant was 75 and 72 per cent for the control and experimental groups, respectively. No statistical difference was found in the parameters studied for either group. The submerged and non-submerged techniques provide similar conditions for osseointegration when two-stage implants are used.

Van Winkelhoff *et al.*[5] \ in 2000, evaluated implant colonisation in partially edentulous patients and the prevalence of periodontal pathogens in the pre- and post-operative periods. Twenty patients, with no clinical signs of caries or periodontitis, who required implant-supported fixed partial dentures of two to three elements in the upper or lower molar and premolar regions were selected. Implants with a diameter of 5 mm were placed according to the Bránemark technique. After 6 months of healing, prosthetic abutments were connected. Nine and 11 prostheses were placed in the mandible and maxilla, respectively. The condition of the gingival tissues was analysed at 1, 6 and 12 months. Radiographs were taken at control and after 12 months. Biological samples were taken before and during the surgical phase and after the implants were loaded. The preoperative analysis included bacteriological assessment of saliva and the deepest sulcus of the oral cavity. Examinations such as plaque index, gingival bleeding and periodontal probing were also carried out. During reopening, sterilised paper cones were used to check the internal surface of the implants for bacteria. One month after the prostheses were installed, samples were taken from the same sites selected preoperatively and from around the implants at 6 and 12 months. The presence of microorganisms was found: *Actinobacillus actinomycetemcomitans, Porphyromonas gingivallis, Prevotella intermédia, Bacteroides forsythus, Fusubacterium nucleatum, Peptostreptococcus micros* and *Campylobacter rectus.* Twenty patients took part in the study. The average plaque index was 0.37; sulcus depth was 4.6 mm; gingival bleeding index was 0.64. Loss of osseointegration was found in one patient, who initially had 50% of *P. gingivallis* detected around the implant at 6 and 12 months. Another patient showed marked loss

bone and two fistulas in 2 implants with a low prevalence of *P. gingivallis* (0.08%). *Fusubacterium nucleatum* and *Prevotella intermédia* were the most commonly found microorganisms in the patients' gingival sulci. *P. gingivallis* and *Actinobacillus actinomycetemcomitans* were found in 3 patients. The relationship between saliva and the subgingival region was weak for most microorganisms. In nine patients, samples from inside the implant revealed a detectable number of bacteria, such as *Fusubacterium nucleatum, P. micros, P. intermédia* and *B. forsythus*. After one month, 60, 90 and 85 per cent of *P. intermédia, P. micros and F. nucleatum* were detected adjacent to the implants, respectively. At six months, the prevalence of these microorganisms in the periodontal sulci around the implants showed the same characteristics, demonstrating a balance in the periodontal flora.

Hermann *et al.*[28] , in 2001, evaluated changes in bone Christianity around implants with welded or two-stage prosthetic abutments by varying the size of the microgap. Six different types of 7mm long implant were analysed and the apical part (SLA) of each implant was sandblasted and treated with $HCl/H_2 SO_4$, determining two types of roughness, 20-40 or 2-4µm. For types A, B and C, a 3 mm high prophetic abutment was laser-welded prior to the experiment, with a micro-gap at the interface of < 10µm (type A), 50 µm (type B) and 100 µm (type C), and they were placed using the non-submerged technique. In types D, E and F, the prosthetic abutments were screwed into two-stage implants, placed according to the non-submerged technique. The micro slit was < 10 µm (type D), 50 µm (type E) and 100 µm (type F). All micro slits were placed 1 mm above the bone crest. Six implants were placed in dog mandibles six months after the extraction of four premolars and the first mandibular molars. After 3 months, the animals were sacrificed and the bone segments with the implants immersed in 4% formaldehyde solution combined with 1% calcium chloride for histological analysis. The specimens were dehydrated and embedded in methylmethacrylate. Mesio-distal and bucco-lingual sections were obtained and stained with toludine blue. The images were analysed and the distance between the microgroove and the first bone contact on the implant was analysed for each implant. Different degrees of peri-implantitis were observed, with types D-F exhibiting a moderate to severe degree and types A-C with no or minimal inflammation. Histologically, there was osseointegration in all the specimens evaluated. The results indicated that types A-C showed a smaller distance between the microgroove and the bone crest compared to implants without welding of the prophetic abutment, revealing that the bone crest of these implants is located more apically compared to welded implants. The height of the bone crest was influenced by the possible movement of the screwed implants, but was not influenced by the size of the microcrack.

Quirynen *et al.*[4] \ in 2002, in a review of the literature, warned about the possibility of osseointegrated implants being compromised by the presence of bacteria and the consequent inflammatory reaction. Studies in animals and longitudinal studies in humans indicate that peri-implantitis is characterised by a microbiota comparable to that of periodontitis (predominance of anaerobic Gram-negative bacteria and spirochetes), although there is no proven link between the diseases. To prevent peri-implantitis, some measures should be considered: periodontal health of the remaining teeth in order to prevent the translocation of bacteria, control of peri-implant pockets and the use of abutments with a polished surface. In addition, factors such as poor oral hygiene and smoking increase the risk of peri-implantitis.

King *etal.*[30] , in 2002, carried out a longitudinal study that evaluated the effect of the size of the micro-gap between prosthetic abutment and implant on bone Christianity and the effect of the forces attributed to two-stage implants with a welded or screwed prosthetic abutment. Six different experimental implants with a length of 9 mm and a diameter of 4.1 mm were used in the study. The apical surface of the implants was treated with sandblasting and acid. Implants A, B and C had welded prosthetic abutments and implants D, E and F had screwed prosthetic abutments, representing two-stage implants. The microgaps had the following dimensions: A and D: < 10 µm, B and E: 50 pm, C and F: 100 µm. All implants had the micro slit positioned 1 mm above the alveolar Christian. Four premolars and the first molars were extracted from dogs and, after six months of healing, the implants were positioned using the non-submerged technique. Radiographs were taken after 10 days, as well as over the following three months. The prosthetic abutments were unscrewed and re-screwed four, eight and ten weeks after surgery. The dogs were then sacrificed and the mandibles dissected and immersed in 4% formaldehyde for histological analysis. Linear measurements were taken from the top of the implant to the first bone contact with the implant. All implants remained stable during the study. The welded/screwed effect was statistically significant, while the microcrack and evaluation time effects were non-significant. Welded implants showed less bone loss compared to screwed implants at the one- and two-month evaluation periods. The average bone loss decreased between two and three months for screwed implants while it remained unchanged for welded implants. The results suggested that the stability of the implant/prosthetic abutment assembly played an important role in the level of bone Christianity.

Leonhardt *et al.*[31] , in 2002, carried out a longitudinal study of osseointegrated implants using clinical, radiographic and microbiological tests to assess changes in periodontal health over time. Fifteen patients treated with implants were followed up for ten years. Fifty-seven implants (31 upper and 26 lower) were evaluated. The presence of plaque, sulcus depth and gingival bleeding were the clinical parameters and subgingival bacterial samples were collected. Radiographic images were taken to assess the bone level. The bacteriological samples were cultured in aerobic and anaerobic media. Three implants were lost after the second surgical stage. The success rate was 93.5% in the maxilla and 96.2% in the mandible. The average bone loss was 1.7mm. Seven patients had a positive plaque index. Sixty-one per cent of the implants showed gingival bleeding after probing. Compared to the natural dentition, there was no statistically significant difference in terms of bone loss. At the initial assessment, 53 per cent were positive for *P. gingivallis,* 100 per cent for *P. intermedia* and 27 per cent for *Actinobacillus actinomycetemcomitans.* After ten years, 20 per cent were positive for *P. gingivallis,* 27 per cent for P. *intermedia* and 20 per cent for *Actinobacillus actinomycetemcomitans.* There was a statistically significant difference in the presence of microorganisms when comparing implants and natural dentition. The presence of pathogenic microorganisms does not mean damage to implant treatment. These microorganisms are part of the resident microbiota and can be associated with stable implants.

Todescan *etal.*[49] , in 2002, evaluated the dimensions and relationships of the peri-implant tissues around osseointegrated implants with different depths in the bone. Dog premolars were extracted and after three months three implants from the Brânemark system were placed on each side of the mandible in three different positions: in group 1 (G1), the implant neck was positioned 1 mm above the bone level; in group 2 (G2), implants positioned at the bone level; in group 3 (G3), implants positioned approximately 1 mm below the bone level. After a healing period of three months, 3 mm high prosthetic abutments were connected to the implants and, after a further three months, the animals were sacrificed, the mandibles extracted and placed in solution for fixation. The following measurements were taken: length of the peri-implant mucosa, length of the junctional epithelium, length of the connective tissue, first contact of the bone on the implant, height of the implant-prosthetic abutment junction and level of the bone crest. Twenty implants were submitted for histological examination. The epithelium was similar in length regardless of implant position. The mean connective tissue lengths were G1: 1.13 mm; G2: 0.92 mm; G3: 1.63 mm, with a difference between G2 and G3. The bone contact surface was 46% for G1, 53.7% for G2 and 49% for G3, with no differences between the groups. The heights of the mucosa and connective tissue were greater when the implants were placed at the level of and below the Christian bone, but the epithelium was similar for all the implants evaluated. There was no increase in bone loss when the microfissure between implant and prosthetic abutment was located below the Christian bone.

Broggini *et al*™, in 2003, evaluated the influence of implant connection time (submerged or non-submerged technique) or the presence of a micro-gap (two-stage implants, non-submerged technique vs. one-stage implants, non-submerged technique) on the composition of inflammatory cells adjacent to the implant. Three types of implant (two-stage, submerged technique; two-stage, non-submerged technique; one-stage, non-submerged technique) were placed in the mandible of dogs. For the implants that were placed using the submerged technique, the prosthetic abutments were removed and re-placed at weeks four, eight and ten. After six months, the dogs were sacrificed and the tissue prepared for histological evaluation. In each 0.00825 mm^2 , mononuclear cells and neutrophils were counted and the cell density calculated. A considerable amount of cells concentrated in the region of the implant-prosthetic abutment interface was found in the two-stage implants, with a gradual decrease in both the apical and coronal directions. In contrast, few cells were found in the tissue adjacent to the one-stage implants, with a statistically significant difference. Cell distribution was similar when the submerged and non-submerged techniques were compared, with a prevalence of neutrophils. A greater number of mononuclear cells were found in the two-stage implants. Bone loss adjacent to one-stage implants was lower compared to two-stage implants. According to the authors, the presence of the implant-prosthetic abutment interface increased the accumulation of inflammatory cells and bone loss.

Piattelli *et al.*[37] , in 2003, carried out a histological evaluation of 2-stage implants placed in monkeys. In a previous study, 108 implants were installed in monkeys and the bone response was evaluated in three situations: delayed loading, immediate loading and immediate installation after extraction. The authors chose 40 of them, installed in the mandible, for the evaluation of this study. They observed resorption at three levels of implant positioning in relation to Christian bone: 1 to 2 mm above (G1 - 15 implants); at level (G2 - 12 implants) and 1 to 1.5 mm below (G3 - 13 implants). Bone growth in the coronal direction (0.13±0.12mm) was observed in G1. Vertical resorption in the apical direction was observed in the other groups (G2 - 2 to 2.1±0.29mm and G3 - 3.6±0.46mm). The three groups differed statistically. According to the authors, the data obtained showed that the location of the microgap at the interfaces between the abutments and implants influences bone resorption, with the most favourable situation being found in those located distant in a coronal direction from the bone Christian. Bone remodelling was not dependent on the three surgical situations: delayed loading, immediate loading and immediate installation after extraction.

Norton[34] , in 2006, evaluated the bone loss of implants located in the posterior region in relation to the junction between the implant and the prosthetic abutment. Patients who received 4.5 mm diameter implants, with the interface between the abutment and the implant positioned at the level of the bone Christian, between 1997 and 2003, were evaluated. Radiographs were taken and bone loss assessed. A total of 181 implants were evaluated in 54 patients. Seventy-three per cent of the implants were placed using the non-submerged technique. Twenty patients received bone grafting prior to implantation. After 12 months, the success rate was 99.4 per cent. Eighty implants in the maxilla and 93 in the mandible were analysed for bone loss. For the maxilla, the average bone loss was 0.56 mm, compared to 0.7 mm for the mandible. The frequency of bone loss was 23.1 per cent in the maxilla and 16.7 per cent of implants in the mandible. The frequency of implants losing more than 1 mm was 25% in the maxilla and 36% in the mandible. There was no difference in bone loss between women and men, or between smokers and non-smokers. There was greater bone loss in the distal region compared to the mesial region.

Quirynen *et al.*[43] in 2006 carried out a prospective study comparing, in partially edentulous patients, the maturation of the microbiota in the peri-implant grooves with subgingival plaque on teeth in the same quadrant at different times by means of DNA hybridisation or PCR. Forty-two partially edentulous patients who had previously received at least two two-stage Brânèmark implants were selected. Most of them had treated chronic moderate gingivitis or periodontitis. Two, four, 13, 26 and 78 weeks after the installation of the prosthetic abutments, biofilm samples were taken from around the implants and from the teeth in the same quadrant. For each patient, samples were taken from four different locations: grooves around implants with a depth of less than 3mm; with a depth greater than 3mm; grooves around teeth with a depth of less than 4mm or greater than 4mm. In addition, clinical indices such as the presence of biofilm, sulcus depth and bleeding after probing were recorded. The samples were evaluated using DNA hybridisation, PCR and bacterial culture. Periodontal parameters did not differ statistically when the shallow grooves of teeth and implants were compared. For grooves with medium or high depth, however, the scores were higher around the teeth. Most of the parameters did not vary over time, with high scores for the deep grooves. DNA hybridisation identified that the microorganisms found in the samples from the shallow grooves around the teeth were similar to those in the peri-implant grooves. For the medium-depth grooves around the teeth, the presence of microorganisms was greater. The difference between teeth and implants was small, regardless of groove depth and evaluation time. An increase in the number of microorganisms was observed over time: *for the* bacteria *F. nucleatum, T. forsythia* and *P. gingivallis* there was an increase in the second and fourth weeks, but not in the thirteenth week. After the second week, the microbiota of the newly created peri-implant grooves already had a complex microbiota. The number of pathogenic microorganisms in the tooth and implant grooves showed a weak correlation between tooth and implant in the second and fourth weeks, but after the thirteenth week, the number was similar. After 26 weeks, the number was identical for implants and teeth with narrow and moderate grooves. In the second week, the implants had a lower frequency compared to the teeth. Three months after prosthetic abutment connection, the presence of *P. gingivallis, A.Actinommycetemcomitans, P. intermedia* and *C. rectus* showed comparable scores between tooth and implant for the shallow grooves. After 18 months, the amount around the implants increased, becoming comparable to teeth with moderate depth grooves. The study indicated that bacteria associated with periodontitis can colonise peri-implant grooves within a week.

Pongnarisorn *et al*[39] in 2007 investigated the nature of the inflammatory reaction in the peri-implant tissue around implants (Nobel Biocare) with abutments of different surfaces. Pathogenic microorganisms were identified. The lower premolars of dogs were removed and, after one month, 64 implants were positioned. The abutments had four different types of surface on the transmucosal portion: A) surface conditioned with hydrofluoric and nitric acid; B) machined surface; C) machined surface with a 0.4 mm wide and long groove; D) surface prepared with anionic oxidation. Clinical and radiographic evaluations were carried out monthly. At six months, a gingival biopsy was carried out and the animals sacrificed. The junctional and oral epithelium were used as a reference for assessing the inflammatory infiltrate. The areas of infiltrate were categorised into three grades: Grade 1: areas with sparse inflammatory cells; Grade 2: areas with moderate inflammatory cells; Grade 3: areas with dense inflammatory cells. Mononuclear cells were counted and the percentage was calculated in the epithelial and vascular infiltrates. Tests were carried out to detect the presence of *Actinommycetemcomitans, Tannerella forsythia, Fusubacterium nucleatum,* and *Porphyromonas gingivallis.* The peri-implant tissues around all the prosthetic abutments showed some signs of inflammation. The type C prosthetic abutment showed areas with the greatest amount of inflammation, while the type B prosthetic abutments showed the smallest areas. No other statistically significant differences were found. T cells predominated among the infiltrated cells, followed by B cells. Many macrophages were detected in the lesions, however no differences in cells were found between the abutments tested. All the dogs showed *Phorhyromonas gingivallis, Fusobacterium nucleatum* and *Tannerella forsythia,* and no *Actinobacillus actinomycetemcomitans. Phorhyromonas gingivallis* was not detected in the type C implants. In most samples, a moderate level of bacteria was found. The results showed that inflammation did not depend on the surface; however, the presence of a sulcus could be associated with larger infiltrates.

2.4 Infiltration at the interface between abutment and implant

Traversy and Birek[50] conducted a study in 1992 to determine whether fluid infiltration at the interfaces between abutments and implants was bidirectional and whether bacteria *(Streptococcus Sanguis)* penetrated between the components of the Branemark implant system. Eight abutment/implant assemblies were immersed in paranitrophenol (PNP) solution and after 24 hours the samples were opened to measure the amount of PNP inside the implants using a spectrophotometer. Eight samples immersed in solution without PNP served as controls and 7 with the interface sealed served as positive controls. In this experiment (infiltration from the outside to the inside of the implant) there was a significant difference ($p< 0.0001$) between the test (0.08 ± 0.002) and control groups (0.01 ± 0.002). In the reverse experiment (infiltration from inside to outside the implant) the differences were again significant (0.390 ± 0.04 vs 0.01 ± 0.01). In the assessment of bacterial infiltration, contamination in both directions was evaluated by counting colony-forming units (CFU) after culturing samples obtained from the respective surfaces of the abutment/implant assemblies using sterile paper cones. A quantity

≥ 10 CFU was considered positive for contamination. Bacterial infiltration occurred in both directions. The authors concluded that bidirectional infiltration of fluids and bacteria occurs through the interfaces between abutments and implants.

In 1993, Quirynen and van Steenberghe[42] carried out an *in vivo* study to investigate the presence of mycoorganisms on the inside of Brànemark implants. The study involved 9 volunteer patients with implants installed more than 2 years previously, no bone resorption, a sulcus depth of 3.5mm around the implant, no antibiotics administered in the 6 months prior to the study and good gingival conditions. Three patients were totally edentulous and 6 were partially edentulous. Two implants were assessed per patient. To assess the presence of bacteria inside the implants, each abutment screw was carefully removed and the apical part was vigorously agitated in sterile 0.85% sodium chloride solution. Special attention was paid to preventing contact between the coronal portion of the screw and the sterile solution. All the samples contained enough microorganisms to be counted. The presence of mainly cocci (86%±8%) and non-motile bacilli (12.3%) was observed. Organisms with motility (1.3%±1.8%) or spirochetes (0.1%) were recorded sporadically. The authors considered that the most likely origin of this contamination could be bacterial infiltration at the interface between the abutment and the implant.

In 1994, Quirynen *et al.*[40] evaluated *in vitro the* existence of bacterial infiltration at the interfaces of Brànemark system implant components. Thirty-two implant/prosthetic abutment/prosthetic crown assemblies were installed in a culture medium previously contaminated with microorganisms. Sixteen assemblies were partially submerged and sixteen completely submerged in the culture medium. After seven days of incubation, the microorganisms from the inside of the components were collected and cultivated in the appropriate culture medium. Microorganisms were found in all the assemblies fully submerged in contaminated culture medium and low contamination was found in the partially submerged assemblies, indicating that there was infiltration in all the conditions tested.

In 1996, Persson *et al.*[38] examined the microbiota on the internal surface of 28 Brànemark implants (Nobelpharma, Sweden) in an *in vivo* study. Ten partially edentulous patients took part in the study, each with a fixed prosthesis supported by 2 to 4 implants that had been in place for 1 to 8 years. A total of 28 implants were evaluated. Two patients had aestheticone abutments and the other 8 had *standard* abutments. The prostheses were checked for mobility and removed. The abutment screws were removed and classified as: stable, easy to remove and loose. Bacteria samples were then taken from the inner surface of the implants. The marginal bone level, mesial and distal, around the implants was measured by means of radiographic evaluations, using radiographs taken immediately after the prostheses were installed. The predominant species were estimated and identified on blood agar plates. Identification was based on Gram staining, oxygen sensitivity and biochemical tests. The internal surfaces of the different components of the Brànemark implants, after varying periods of function in the oral cavity, harboured a heterogeneous and anaerobic microbiota. The individual samples showed great variation. No relationship could be established between the type and length of the abutment, the stability of the abutment, bone loss, type and number of microorganisms

found in the samples. The flora consisted mainly of facultative and anaerobic *streptococcus*, Gram-positive and anaerobic bacilli such as *Propionibacterium, Eubacterium* and *Actinomyces,* as well as anaerobic Gram-negative bacilli including *Fusobacterium, Prevotella* and *Porphyromonas.* For the authors, there are reasons to suggest that this presence of bacteria is the result of contamination of the components during the 1^2 and 2^2 surgical stages of implant and abutment installation and/or the transmission of microorganisms from the oral cavity during the function and subsequent installation of the prosthesis.

Jansen *et al.*[29] , in 1997, evaluated microbial penetration at the interface between the abutment and the implant and correlated the size of the interface and the amount of infiltration. Thirteen different prophetic implant-abutment combinations (Ankylos, Degussa Dentsply - conical connection solid abutment; Astra, Astra Tech - conical connection solid abutment; Bonefit, Strauman - conical connection solid abutment; Bonefit, Strauman - slightly angled octagonal socket connection abutment and screw; Brànemark, Nobel Biocare - flat connection abutment and screw; Calcitec, - flat connection abutment and screw; Frialit-2, Dentsply Friadent - flat connection abutment and screw with silicone ring; Ha-Ti, Mathis Dental Implants - initially flat connection abutment and screw and tapered at the bottom; Ha-Ti, Mathis Dental Implants - flat connection abutment and screw; IMZ - flat connection abutment and screw; IMZ, IMZ implants - solid flat connection abutment; Semados - slightly angled solid flat connection abutment) were subjected to microbiological testing. The internal parts of the implants were filled with *Escherichia coli.* The assembly was then immersed up to a few millimetres above the interface in a tube containing nutrient solution and possible penetration on days 1, 3, 5, 7, 10 and 14. The implant-prosthetic abutment interface was measured using SEM in each combination. The Calcitek implant and the Ha-Ti system showed bacterial infiltration under all conditions. The application of the silicone ring reduced microleakage. In most cases, infiltration was observed within the first two days. All the conical prosthetic abutments had a tapered interface. The interfaces were less than 10 µm in all cases.

Guindy et a/.[26] , in 1998, investigated bacterial microleakage between Ha-Ti implants,

Mathis Dental Implants, and prefabricated crowns in the marginal gap and screw region. The Ha-Ti implant components consist of an implant, prosthetic abutment, axial screw, prefabricated alloy crown and transverse screw. Thirty prefabricated crowns were divided into three groups depending on their thickness: 3-5mm, 60-72mm and 114-136mm. Each of the specimens was incubated in a test tube containing 3ml of *S. aureus* in TSB medium and removed at intervals between 24 and 120 hours. After removal from the culture medium, paper tips were used to take samples from inside the alloy crown and the prosthetic abutment. Each paper tip was incubated in tubes containing TSB medium. The growth of *S. aureus* was recorded after 24 hours. In the second experiment, the internal hexagon of each implant was inoculated in culture, then the prosthetic abutment was placed in position and screwed in place. A new culture was injected through the screw hole after the crown was joined to the prosthetic abutment with the transverse screw. Each specimen was incubated in 3 ml of TSB medium and the growth of the bacteria recorded after 24 hours. The experiments were carried out under two conditions: with the crown-implant assembly fully immersed in medium or partially immersed (up to the implant/prosthetic abutment interface). Bacterial infiltration was found for all three groups when the specimens were completely immersed for 24-48 hours. For the partially immersed groups, bacterial growth was recorded at all times. Bacterial infiltration occurred through the transverse screw, not through the marginal microcrack of the prefabricated crowns.

Besimo *et al.*[5] , in 1999, evaluated the sealing capacity to prevent bacterial infiltration in Ha-Ti implants, Mathis Dental Implants, and prefabricated crowns. Ha-Ti implants use prosthetic abutments and prefabricated noble alloy crowns. Thirty prefabricated crowns with a diameter of 4.5 mm were used. To check for infiltration inside the specimens, a 1% chlorhexidine varnish was applied to all contact surfaces of the implant components. The crown was fixed to the implant and the assembly immersed in culture for *S. aureus* in plastic tubes. Initially, the assembly was completely immersed for eight weeks, then the assembly was partially immersed (up to the microcrack) for a further 11 weeks. Samples were then taken with paper tips from the inner region of the crown and the inner hexagon of the implant. The paper tips were swabbed in culture medium and incubated for 24 hours. In a second test, a sample of the bacteria was injected into the implant hexagon before the prosthetic abutment was screwed into place. Next, a new bacterial collection was inserted into the prosthetic abutment before the crown was screwed into place. The assembly was then immersed in culture medium for one week. Bacterial growth was recorded. Bacterial infiltration was found in one of the five fully immersed specimens after four weeks, and was not detected at 3, 5, 6, 7 or 8 weeks. When the specimens were partially submerged between 13 and 11 weeks, no infiltration was observed. Chlorhexidine proved effective in reducing microleakage between implant components.

Gross *et al.*[25] , in 1999, evaluated the degree of microleakage of fluids at the interface between the abutment and the implant of 5 systems available on the market, varying the torque. The implant systems tested were: Spline (Sulzer), ITI (Straumann), CeraOne (Nobel), Steri-Oss (Steri-Oss) and
3i (Implant Innovations). Each implant was sectioned in the apical region and a channel was prepared from the apex to the base of the screw. Torques were set at 10, 20 N or according to each manufacturer. The implants were inserted into pressure-controlled silicone tubes, sealed with thread and filled with low molecular weight dye. Fluid passage at the interface between the abutment and the implant was measured at different times. A gradual increase in microleakage occurred over time for all implant systems. Microleakage decreased significantly with increasing torque and was system-dependent at twenty minutes, with ITI showing the greatest infiltration. At the other assessment times, infiltration was similar for all systems.

Rimondinni *et al.*[45] conducted an *in vivo* study *in* 2001 to investigate internal microbial contamination in implants with screw-retained abutments. The assemblies evaluated were in function in the mouth, subjected to occlusal loads with cemented provisional restorations. They evaluated the effect of using a silicone ring at the interface between the abutment and the implant. Seven patients with perfect oral hygiene participated in the study, in which 8 implants had silicone rings and 7 did not. After 2 months in place, the provisional crowns and abutment screws were removed and the organic and inorganic contamination of the screws was examined by scanning electron microscopy (SEM) and energy dispersive spectroscopy (EDS). Amorphous and crystalline contamination, suggestive of calcium and phosphate components, was found in all abutment screws and the presence of bacteria was more frequently observed in the group without the silicone ring. No difference was observed in the types of bacteria in the sealed and unsealed groups. The presence of *coccus* was more representative and *bacillus was* less common. According to the authors, in clinical situations, infiltration occurs at the interfaces between abutments and implants, but this contamination is limited in patients with good oral hygiene and can be reduced with the use of the silicone ring.

Piattelli *et al.*[36] , in 2001, evaluated the penetration of fluids and bacteria and two implant systems: cemented prosthetic abutment or screwed prosthetic abutment. Twelve cemented or screwed implants were immersed in dye and culture medium previously contaminated with microorganisms and examined using SEM, and the penetration of fluids and bacteria assessed. The SEM observations revealed that there is a gap of two to seven micrometres in the screw-retained abutments, while for the cement-retained abutments, the gap is seven micrometres, completely filled by the cement. In the screw-retained abutments, the presence of dye was detected in all implants at the abutment/implant interface and inside the implants, as well as the presence of bacteria, and there was no infiltration of dye or bacteria inside the implants with the cemented abutments. Cemented abutments showed better infiltration results compared to screw-retained abutments.

Cravinhos[15] , in 2003, assessed the quality and precision of the implant/prosthetic connector interface in 3 surgical 2-stage implant systems available on the Brazilian market, by means of an *in vitro* microbiological assessment. For this purpose, 30 implants were used, divided into 3 groups of 10 units, group 1 being those belonging to the Colosso® system, group 2 to the Conect® system and group 3 to the Globtek® system. After handling and opening the implants under sterile conditions, 0.1 µL of a solution containing a colony of *Streptococcus sanguis* bacteria was inoculated onto the inner surface of each implant and, immediately afterwards, the prosthetic connector was adapted and screwed in using a torque wrench calibrated at 30 Nem. The implant/prosthetic connector composition was then placed in a container containing BHI (Brain Heart Infusion) culture medium and taken to a bacteriological oven, which was kept under ideal conditions for 14 days, and every 24 hours the presence or absence of visible contamination was observed. All the implant systems used in the study were found to have bacterial microleakage, but no statistically significant differences were observed between the systems evaluated.

Amaral[3] , in 2003, evaluated bacterial contamination through the implant/prosthetic connector interface in an *in vitro* study, seeking to correlate it with the dimensions of the spaces at the interface. 50 implant compositions were used with their respective prosthetic connectors (CONIC® - Group 1, MASTER POROUS® - Group 2, SERSON® - Group 3, INP® - Group 4 and IMPLAC® - Group 5), divided into 5 groups of 10 units. The microbiological analysis was carried out after the *Streptococcus sanguis* bacterium was inoculated into the inside of the implant, followed by the adaptation of a prosthetic connector screwed in manually at a torque of 32 N. The composition was inserted into a BHI *(Brain Heart Infusion)* culture medium stored in a bacteriological oven for 14 days, and a daily reading was taken to check for contamination. After 14 days, the implants were taken for analysis under a scanning electron microscope to check the size of the spaces at the implant/prosthetic connector interface, with magnification ranging from 30 to 2000 X. The results were submitted to the proportion test at a significance level of 5% to compare the percentage of contaminated implants and the sizes of the gaps found. All the groups evaluated showed a high degree of bacterial infiltration at the implant/prosthetic connector interface, with the exception of group 3, which showed a lower result, which was statistically significant in relation to the other groups. There was no correlation between the dimensions of the spaces at the implant/prosthetic connector interface and the bacterial contamination observed in the implant systems studied.

Callan *et al.*[3] , in 2005, used DNA probe analysis to identify periodontopathogenic bacteria that may be present on the inside of implants and prosthetic abutment screws in an *in vivo* study. Thirty-two patients (17 women and 15 men) with a mean age of 55.5 years and excellent periodontal health took part in the study. A total of 54 2-stage implants (24 in the maxilla and 30 in the mandible) from various manufacturers were evaluated. Using sterile paper cones, samples were taken from the internal surfaces of the interfaces on 43 implants and from the abutment screw threads of 11 implants. The samples were submitted to the laboratory of the manufacturer of the DNA probe analysis kit and the following bacteria were evaluated: *Actinobacillus actinomycetemcomitans, Tannerella forsythensis, Campylobacter rectus, Eikenella corrodens, Fusobactterium nucleatum, Porphyromonas gingivallis. Prevotella intermédia and Treponema denticola.* All the samples obtained from the abutment screws (n=11) were negative (less than 0.1% of the total). In contrast, 100 per cent of the samples from the inner portion of the interfaces between the abutments and implants (n=43) were positive for one or more microbes. There was no difference between the colonisation of individual species of microbes when comparing the different implant location regions. The authors concluded that moderate to high levels of 8 different periodontopathogenic microbes inhabit the inside of implants. The microbes colonised these surfaces within 25 days of the second surgical stage. According to the authors, these findings support those of other studies showing the passage of bacteria from the residual dentition to the implants.

Dibart *et al.*[17] in 2005 evaluated the sealing capacity of implants with conical prosthetic abutments against bacterial infiltration *in vitro.* Twenty-five implants (5x11 mm) and 25 prosthetic abutments were divided into two experiments: the implant-prosthetic abutment assembly was immersed in a culture of the bacteria *A. actinomycetemcomitans,*

Streptococcus oralis and Fusobacterium nucleatum for 24 hours. The implants were then prepared for evaluation by SEM. In the second experiment, a quantity of bacteria was inserted into the prosthetic abutments, which were placed in position on the implant. A negative control, without the insertion of bacteria, and a positive control, without the insertion of the prosthetic abutment into the implant, were carried out. The implant-prosthetic abutment assembly was inserted into tubes containing culture medium and kept for 72 hours. Then, 20 µL were removed from inside the implant and cultured again for five days. On SEM observation, the authors could see that the bacteria adhered only to the external bevelled part of the prosthetic abutment. The presence of the bacteria ceases approximately 200 pm around the implant-prosthetic abutment junction. In the second experiment, the control group had polluted broth, which means bacterial growth. The other groups showed no contamination of the culture medium. The lack of bacterial invasion reveals the strong sealing capacity of conical implants.

Steinebrunner *et al.*[47] , in 2005, evaluated bacterial infiltration at the implant-prosthetic abutment interface in new implant systems. Five different components were evaluated: Brånemark (Nobel), Frialit-2 (Dentsply), Replac Select (Nobel), Camlog (Altatec) and Screw Vent (Zimmer). Prosthetic abutments for crowns cemented with an anti-rotational system were selected. Each implant was embedded in acrylic resin. Metal crowns were made for each prosthetic abutment and cemented with Panavia 21 (Kuraray). The implants were autoclaved and the inside filled with a suspension of *Escherichia coli* bacteria.
The prosthetic abutment-crown assembly was then connected to the implant. The specimens were then partially immersed in nutrient solution and mechanically cycled (120N, 1200000 cycles, 1 Hz). The solution was placed in a new culture medium for 24 h, and bacterial growth associated with microleakage. All specimens showed bacterial infiltration. The Camlog system showed greater bacterial infiltration than the Frialit and Screw Vent systems. The number of infiltration-free cycles was 17,2800 for the Brånemark system, 43,200 for Frialit, 6,4800 for Replace and 24,300 for Screw Vent.

Covani *et al.*™ in 2006 examined the distribution of bacteria on the internal and external surfaces of failed implants using histological analysis. Ten pure titanium and 5 hydroxyapatite-coated implants were removed from 7 patients. The criteria for removal were peri-implant radiolucency and clinical mobility. The abutments were kept in the implants during removal in order to observe bacteria at the interfaces and on the implant surfaces. After appropriate treatment, the samples were embedded in epoxy resin and sectioned into

4 slices for microscopic observation. Radiographs were taken and showed the presence of a thin radiolucent space in all the implants. All the abutments were well fixed to the implants. Histological examination showed the presence of microbiota, epithelial cells and fibrous tissue around the implants. Filaments, bacilli, fusiforms and spirochetes were present without any orientation, forming layers of different thicknesses between the implants and the soft tissue. High bacterial colonisation was observed at the interface level between the abutments and implants. For the authors, this may legitimise the hypothesis that the microfissure formed at this interface at bone level may present a risk of bone loss.

Dias[16] , in 2007, assessed maladaptation at the interface between the implant and its respective prosthetic abutment in six systems manufactured and marketed in Brazil, and verified bacterial infiltration through this interface. To assess maladaptation, five samples of each system were tested: Neodent Titamax, Neodent Cone Morse, Titanium Fix, Conexão, SIN and Dentoflex, to which the torques recommended by the manufacturers were applied. Maladaptation measurements were taken at 12 equidistant points using scanning electron microscopy at magnifications of up to 20,000 times. In the second stage of the experiment, eight sets of each system were inoculated with 0.5μl of a suspension containing *Escherichia coli to* analyse bacterial infiltration. The samples were analysed after inoculation at 24h, 48h, on the 5th° , 7th° , and 14th day, by observing the turbidity of the culture medium. The results showed better adaptation for the Titanium Fix system (0.113±1.774μm), followed by the Neodent Titamax (0.852±0.639μm), Dentoflex (0.927±2.329μm), Conexão (1.319±1.600μm), SIN (2.301 ±1.774μm) and Neodent Cone Morse (3.232±2.821μm) systems. The system that showed bacterial infiltration in the largest number of samples was the Neodent Cone Morse, with all eight samples (100%), while the Dentoflex system showed bacterial infiltration in seven samples (87.5%), Titanium Fix and Conexão showed infiltration in five samples (62.5%), SIN and Neodent Titamax showed infiltration in one sample (12.5%). In this study it was not possible to establish a relationship between the size of the maladaptation and bacterial infiltration.

In 2007, Santana[46] evaluated the micro-infiltration of the interface between abutments and implants of prosthetic connections with internal hexagon and cone morse systems. The study selected 35 implants divided into 7 groups (5 groups of implants from domestic companies and 2 groups from imported companies). The foreign implants tested were Straumann (Straumann AG® / Switzerland), Ankylos (Dentsply-Friadent® / Germany), while the domestic implants were AR Morse (Conexão/Sistema de Prótese® Sào Paulo-SP), Titamax CM (Neodent® / Curitiba-PR), Titamax II (Neodent®/Curitiba-PR), Stronger

(Sin/Sistema Nacional de Implante® São Paulo - SP) and Titanium Fix CM (AS Technology / São José dos Campos-SP). For the contamination tests, the bacteria *Enterococcus faecalis* was inoculated inside the implant with immediate installation and torque (N/cm^2) of the respective prosthetic abutment. Subsequently, the abutment/implant set was placed in brain and heart infusion (BHI) broth culture medium and kept in this medium for a period of 14 days. The control was carried out by clouding the culture medium and evaluated for 7 days and 14 days. The results showed that all the samples from the Ankylos and Neodent CM groups did not show microleakage, while 20 per cent of the AR Morse Connection group showed microleakage; however, there were no statistically significant differences when compared to the previous groups. In addition, the Straumann, Titanium-Fix CM, Neodent Plus and SIN Strong group samples all showed infiltration after 14 days of the study (significance level a=0.05) and, when assessing the correlation between these samples, it was found that there were no statistically significant differences.

Do Nascimento *et al.*™, in 2008, investigated the infiltration of *Fusobacterium nucleatum* through the interface between implants and prefabricated and cast external hexagon abutments (n=10) (Sin® system, São Paulo, Brazil). They evaluated the passage of bacteria from inside the implant to the external environment for 14 days. The implants were inoculated with 3pl of bacterial suspension and the abutments connected with a torque of 32Ncm. The top of each sample was sealed with a layer of guttapercha and cyanocrylate adhesive. One sample from each group was eliminated from the study due to immediate external contamination, leaving 9 in each group. Bacterial infiltration was observed in one sample from each group (11.1%). The authors concluded that if the casting instructions and procedures indicated by the manufacturer are followed, prefabricated or cast abutments can show low rates of bacterial infiltration.

Faria *et al.*[23] , in 2008, carried out a pilot study to compare two methodologies, checking external contamination (EC) after inoculation and torque, in three types of abutment/implant connections (n=20): External Hexagon (HE), Indexed Internal Hexagon (HI) and Morse Cone (CM). In methodology 1, 0.7 µl of *Escherichia coli* suspension was inoculated inside the implants and the respective abutments connected with a torque of 20Ncm. In Method 2, an *E. coli colony* was inoculated into the apical portion of the abutment screw before the torque was applied. The assemblies were placed on plates with TSA and covered with liquid agar; after rolling, the plates were taken to a bacteriological oven at 37^9 C to check colony growth after 24 hours. In methodology 1, the percentage of external contamination (%EC) was 5, 60 and 45 per cent for HE, HI and CM, respectively. In methodology 2, the %CE was 10, 5 and 0% for HE, HI and CM, respectively. The authors concluded that the bacterial colony inoculation methodology showed less external contamination during the experiment, resulting in less waste and greater efficiency in data collection.

CHAPTER 3

PROPOSAL

To evaluate the infiltration of *Escherichia coli* at the interfaces between abutments and implants in external hexagon, indexed internal hexagon and Morse cone prosthetic connections.

The null hypotheses of the research will be:

H_0 -i: In the three conditions tested, the interfaces between abutments and implants will remain free of bacterial infiltration.

H -02 : THE different types of connections tested will not differ from each other.

CHAPTER 4

MATERIAL AND METHOD

The project was carried out at the Department of Bioscience and Oral Diagnosis, in the Microbiology laboratory of the São José dos Campos School of Dentistry - UNESP.

To assess bacterial infiltration in three types of prosthetic connections, 150 sets of abutments and implants, 50 for each group, were used.

The different types of abutment-implant combinations (Conexão Sistemas de Prostótese, Brazil) were divided into three groups (n=50) (table 1):

Table 1 - distribution of the groups studied.

Group	Implant	Connection type	Prophetic pillar
G1	Master Screw 4.0/13mm	External hexagon	Preparation pillar + fixing screw
G2	AR Morse 4.0/13mm	Morse cone or indexed internal hexagon	Internal hexagon preparation abutment + fixing screw
G3	AR Morse 4.0/13mm	Morse cone or indexed internal hexagon	Solid microunit abutment (Morse cone)

The AR Morse implant has a double internal configuration and can receive Morse cone or indexed internal hexagon prosthetic abutments. For this reason, the implants in groups G2 and G3 are the same, with only the types of prosthetic abutments differing.

Figure 1 illustrates the three different types of prosthetic connections.

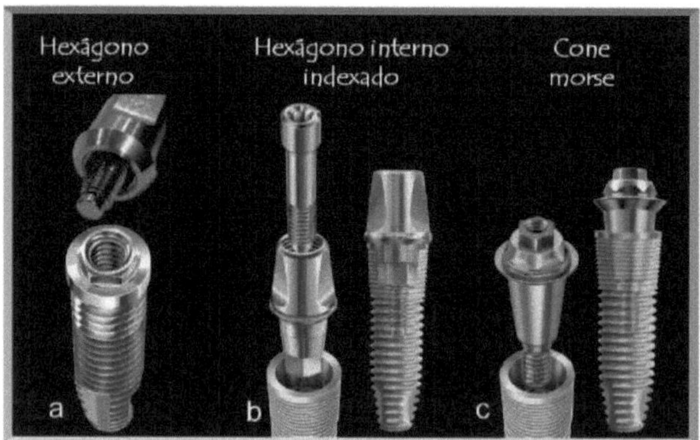

FIGURE 1 - A - Implant and External Hexagon connection abutment; B - Implant and Indexed Internal Hexagon connection abutment; C - Implant and Cone Morse connection abutment.

The technique used to check for bacterial infiltration through the interface between the abutment and the implant was the reverse technique, i.e. the passage of bacteria from inside the implant to the external environment. *Escherichia coli* ATCC 25922 was used

(Figure 2), which was seeded by draining onto plates containing Tryptic Soy Agar (TSA) (Acumedia Manufacters, Inc. Lansing, Michigan). The plates were incubated at 37 ± 1^S C for 24 hours to allow bacterial growth.

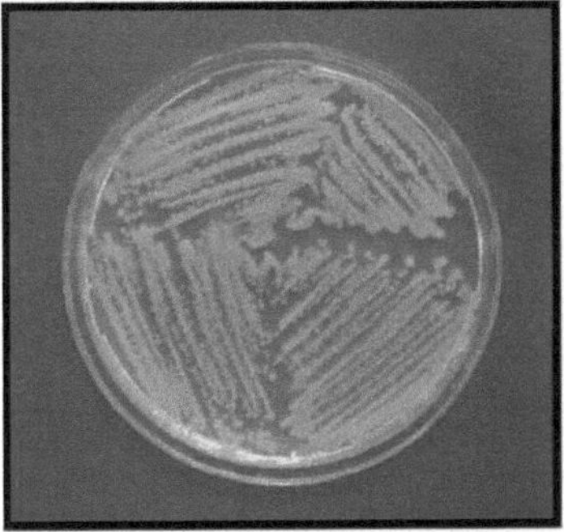

FIGURE 2 - Sowing of *E.coli* by depletion on plates containing TSA.

During the experimental stages, care was taken to avoid contaminating the working field. All procedures were carried out in a sterile environment, inside the laminar flow chamber, which was lined with sterile surgical drapes. All the instruments used were previously sterilised in a steam autoclave (121^9 for 15 minutes) and all the steps were carried out using sterile gloves. The work was carried out by three operators who remained in the same role until the end of the experiment. Two operators kept their clothes on while working in the laminar flow chamber and the third helped to supply the necessary material and record information for the organisation of the research.

Each implant was placed in a sterile vise using sterile forceps, allowing the implant to be properly fixed. Using a platinum needle previously flambéed in a Bunsen burner, part of an isolated colony of *E. coli* was collected and immediately inoculated into the apical portion of the abutment screw (Figures 3 to 6).

After inoculating the bacteria, the abutments were connected, tightened with a torque of 20Ncm to the implants according to the manufacturer's protocol and held for 5 seconds (figures 7 and 8). A manual torque wrench was used (Conexão Sistemas de Prótrese, São Paulo, Brazil).

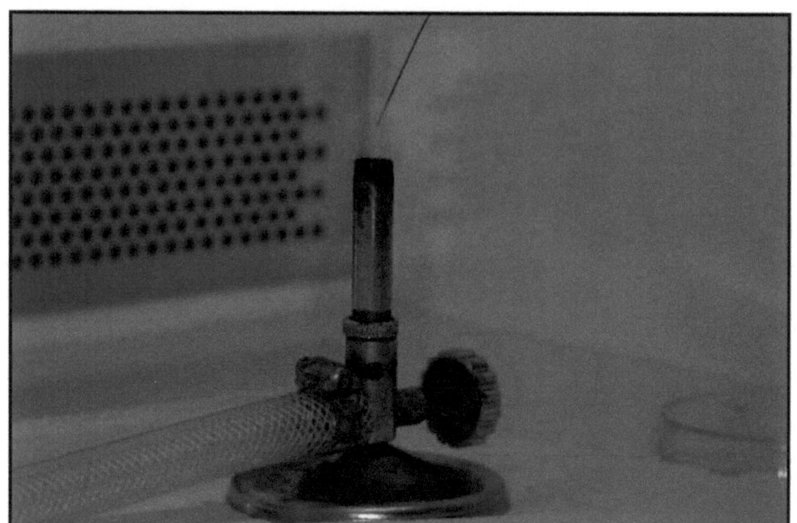

FIGURE 3 - Flamed platinum needle.

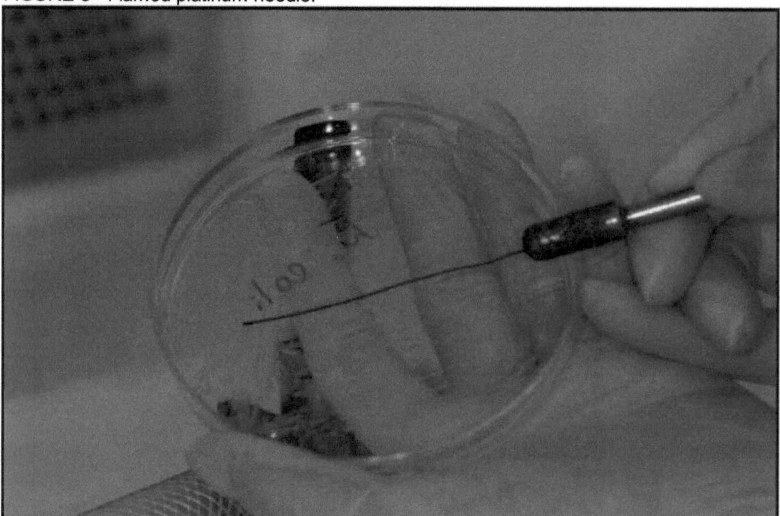

FIGURE 4 - *E. coli colony* collection;

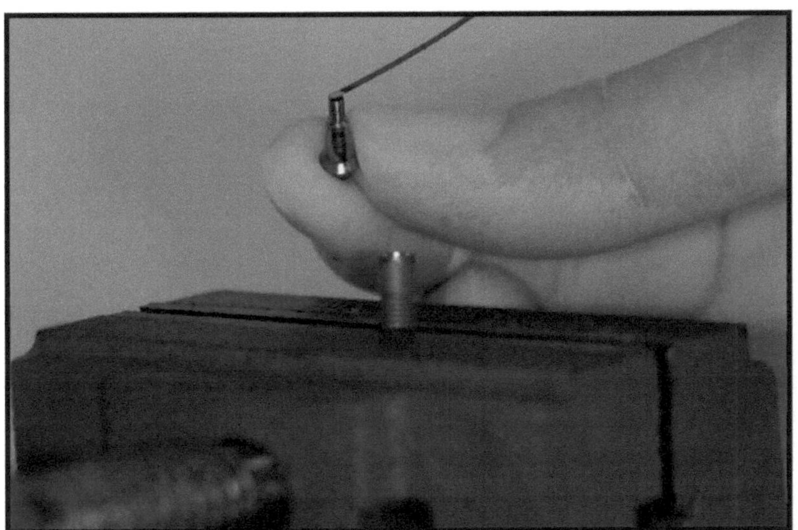

FIGURE 5 -Inoculation of *E. coli in* the apical part of the abutment screw *(cone morse microunit)*.

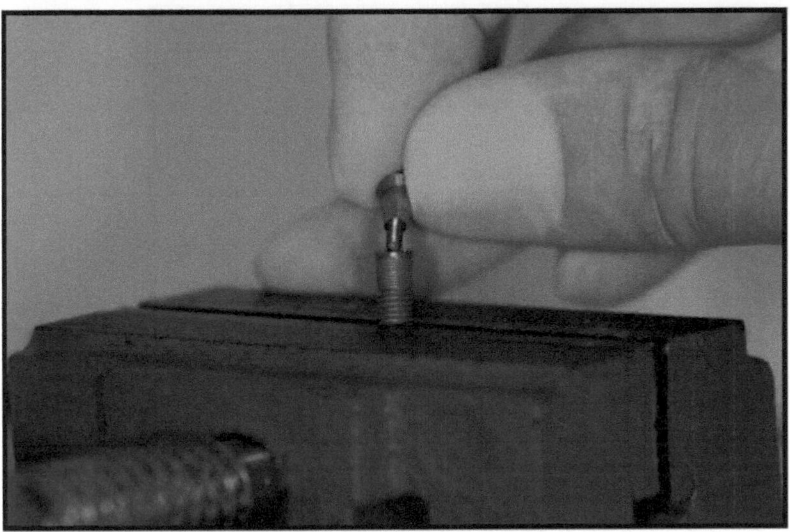

FIGURE 6 - Fitting the abutment to the implant.

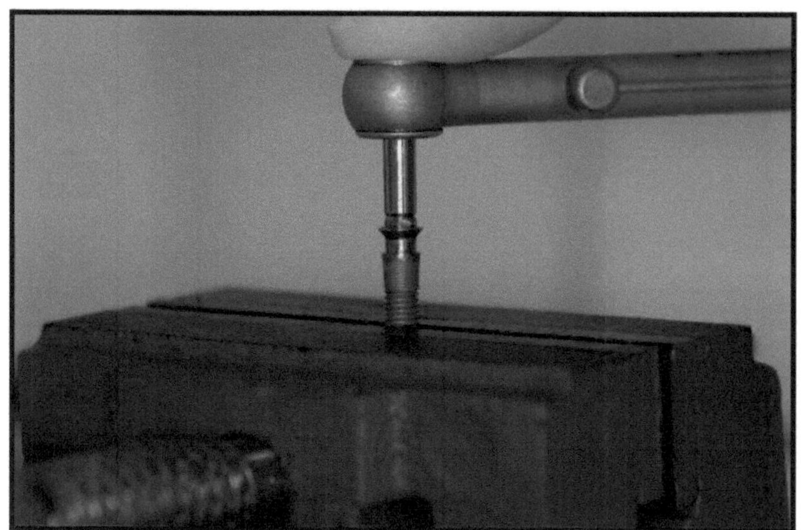
FIGURE 7 - Fitting the relevant spanner and torque wrench.

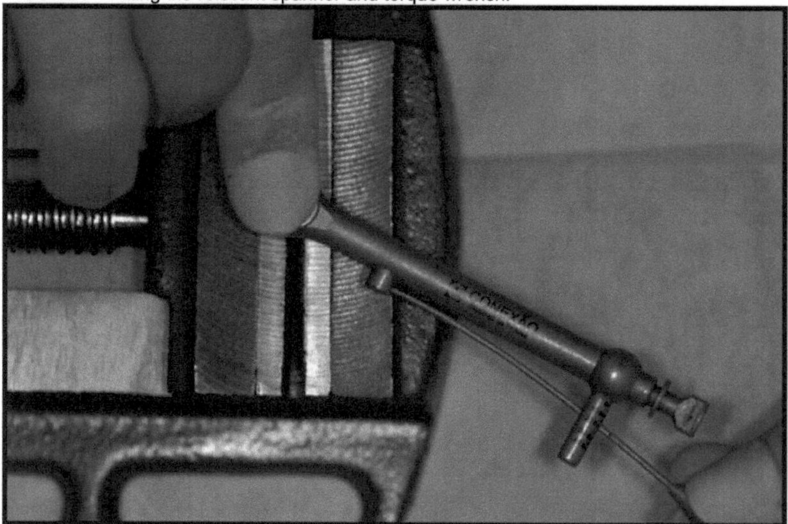
FIGURE 8 - Application of 20 Nem torque for 5 seconds.

To check for possible immediate external contamination during the execution of the methodology, each set, abutment and implant, was rolled in a Petri dish containing TSA, then covered with solubilised agar (TSA) and removed from the dish. Afterwards, each set was placed in a test tube containing 4 mL of Tryptic Soy Broth (TSB) (Acumedia Manufacters, Inc. Lansing, Michigan) (figures 9 to 14). The plates with solidified agar were incubated at 37°C for 24 hours to check for possible bacterial growth. The sets corresponding to the contaminated plates were discarded from the study.

The samples from groups G1 and G2 (implants with two-part abutments) were suspended and stabilised in the test tube using a special device made manually with 0.30 mm diameter chromium nickel (CrNi) wire (Dental Moreli, Sorocaba), so that only the interface region between the abutment and the implant remained in contact with the culture medium without the possibility of bacteria escaping through the interface between the abutment and the screw (Figures 11 to 14). For the samples in group G3, this procedure was not necessary, as the abutment is solid and there is no other way for bacteria to exit the internal portion of the implant, other than through the interface between the abutment and the implant (Figures 9 and 10).

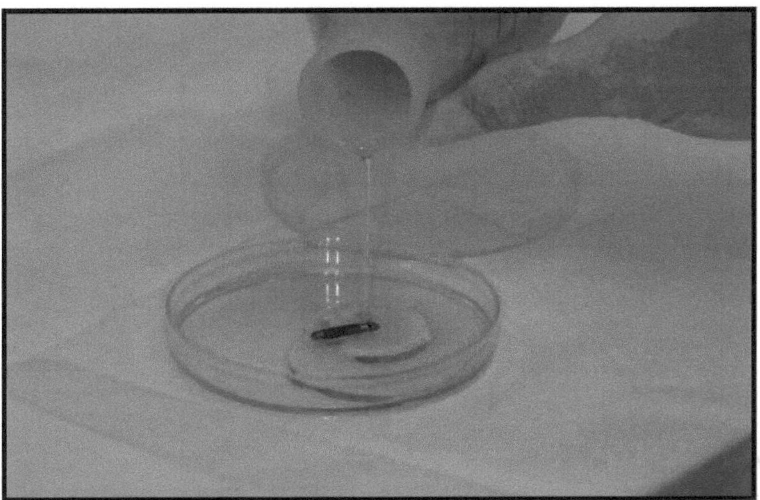

FIGURE 9 - Covering the implant and cone morse abutment assembly with solubilised agar.

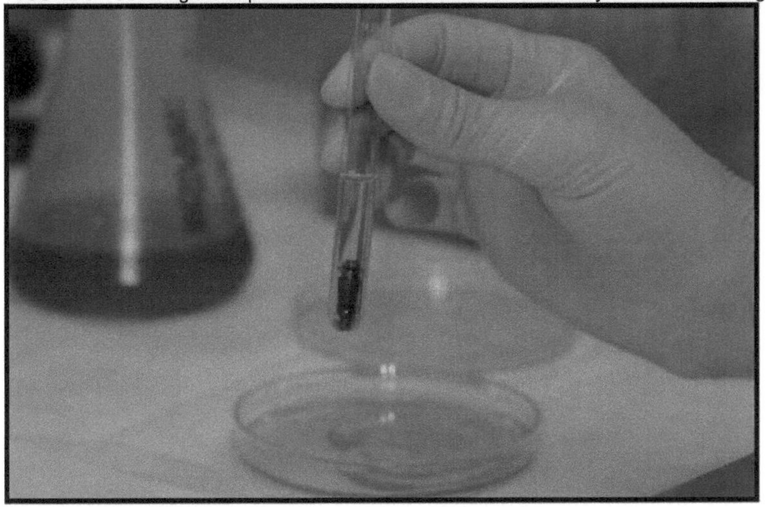

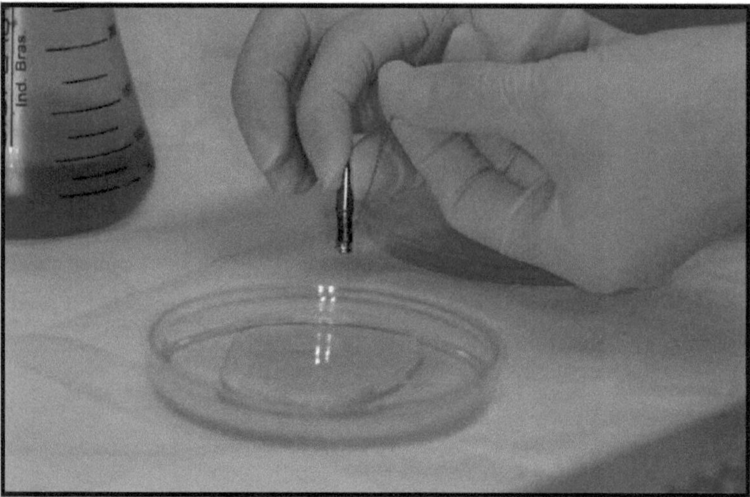

FIGURE 11 - Removal of the implant and indexed internal hexagon abutment assembly from the plate and positioning of the assembly in the metal stabilisation device.

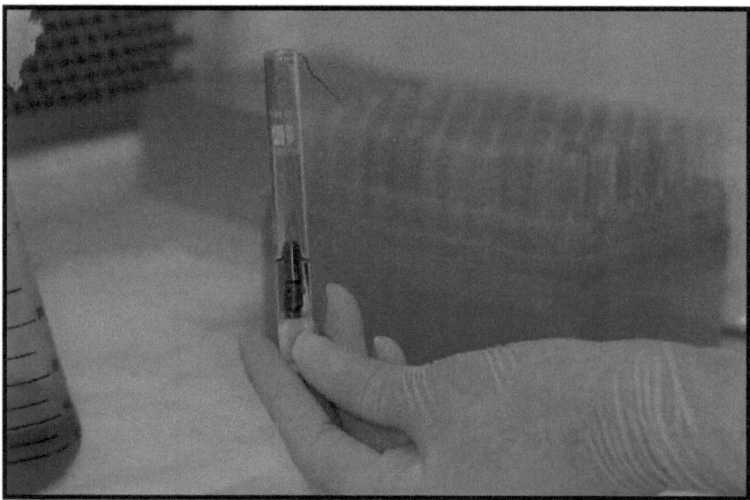

FIGURE 12 - Immersion of the stabilised assembly in the test tube.

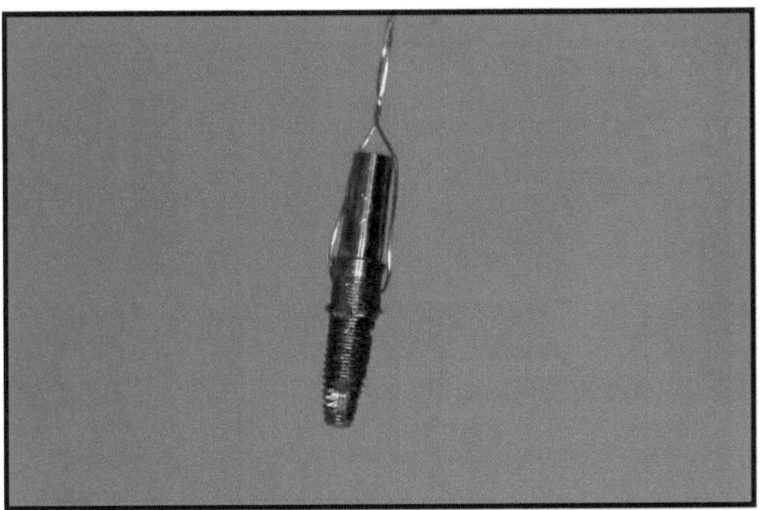

FIGURE 13 - Aspect of the implant and external hexagon abutment assembly immediately after removal of the plaque, stabilised in the metal device.

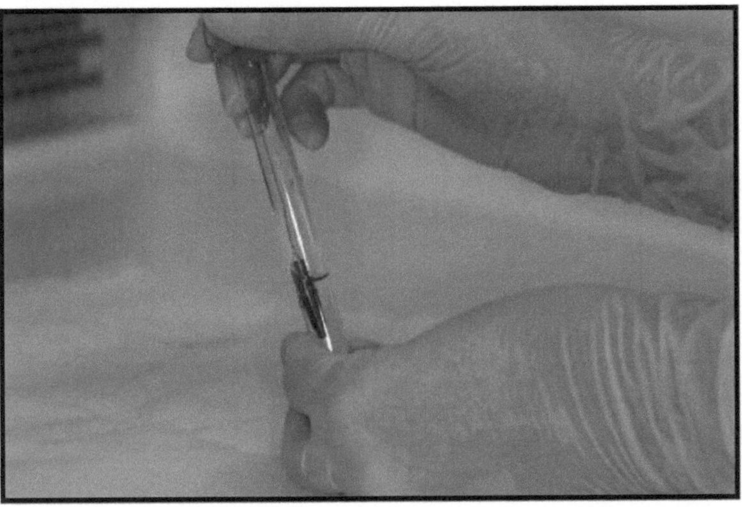

FIGURE 14 - Immersion of the set in a tube containing TSB broth being kept partially immersed.

The appearance of the samples from the three groups in the test tube containing TSB broth is shown in figure 15 A.

All the tubes containing the sets of abutments and implants were numbered, placed on a rack in an upright position and incubated at 37º C (Figure 5 B).

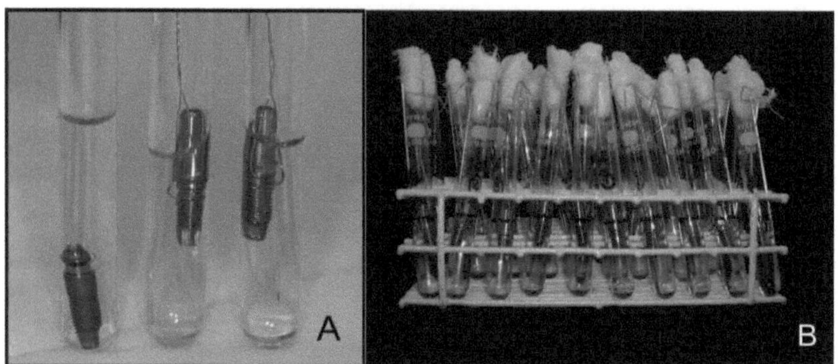
FIGURE 15 - A - Samples from groups G1, G2 and G3 in the test tube containing TSB broth; B - Rack containing the numbered tubes with the different samples.

Daily monitoring was carried out to check for the possible passage of bacteria from inside the implant into the broth. The indication of infiltration through the interface was the turbidity of the culture medium (TSB broth) (Figure 16).

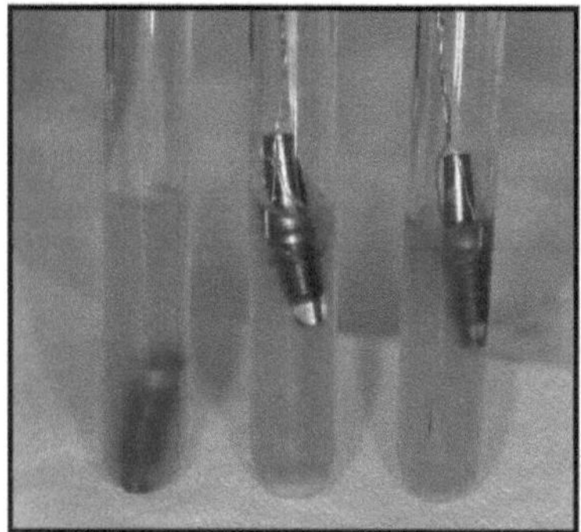
FIGURE 16 - Different specimens that showed turbidity of the culture medium, indicating bacterial infiltration.

In the samples that showed turbidity of the medium, the turbid broth was sown in Petri dishes containing TSA. The plates were incubated at 37°C for 24 hours to observe bacterial growth (E. *coli).* To ensure that only *E. coli was present,* the Gram stain test was carried out on both the cloudy broth and the colonies present on the agar (TSA). The staining and bacterial morphology were observed under an optical microscope. The following procedures were carried out:

- remove a portion of the turbid broth with a sterile platinum loop and place it on a sterile glass slide;

- drying the material placed on the slide;

- fixing

- placing the crystal violet dye on the material and washing the slide after one minute;

46

- placing lugol, a fixative for crystal violet, on the material and washing it off after one minute;

- pour 70% ethyl alcohol on the material and rinse after fifteen seconds;

- placing the fuchsin dye on the material and washing it off after 30 seconds;

- After drying and applying immersion oil, the slide was taken to the optical microscope to observe the colour and bacterial morphology using the immersion lens.

The colonies in the Petri dishes were also Gram-stained after 24 hours of growth in the turbid broth.

The experiments were evaluated over a period of seven days. The evaluation period was determined on the basis of a pilot study in which the implants were opened daily and material was collected from inside them by swabbing with a paper cone and saline solution. The bacteria were found to be viable for seven days.

After this period, in all samples in which there was no turbidity of the medium, the implants were opened in a sterile environment (inside the laminar flow chamber) and the contents of their interior were collected using sterile endodontic paper cones and sterile saline solution, which were rolled in Petri dishes containing TSA. This procedure was carried out to check the viability of the bacteria and the possible efficiency of the seal at the interface between abutment and implant. The seeded plates were kept in a bacteriological oven at 37^S C for 24/48 hours to check for bacterial growth.

Samples that showed immediate external contamination and those that showed neither turbidity nor viability within 7 days were discarded from the study. As a result, the number of samples taken into account when calculating the research results was reduced and is shown in the results.

In addition to analysing bacterial infiltration, 6 sets of abutments and implants of each type of prosthetic connection were evaluated using digital optical microscopy (Mitutoyo, Model AT112-50F, Series 650101, Mitutoyo Corporation, Japan). The assemblies were embedded in resin and sectioned longitudinally for the evaluations. The aim was to illustrate the mechanical relationship between the abutment and the implant. The images are shown in Figures 17 to 19.

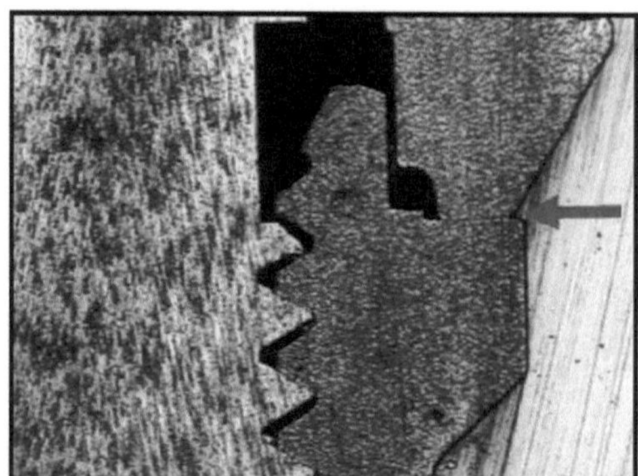

FIGURA 17   - External hexagon connection (gap width at implant/abutment interface =1   .4µm. Optical microscope photograph (63 X).

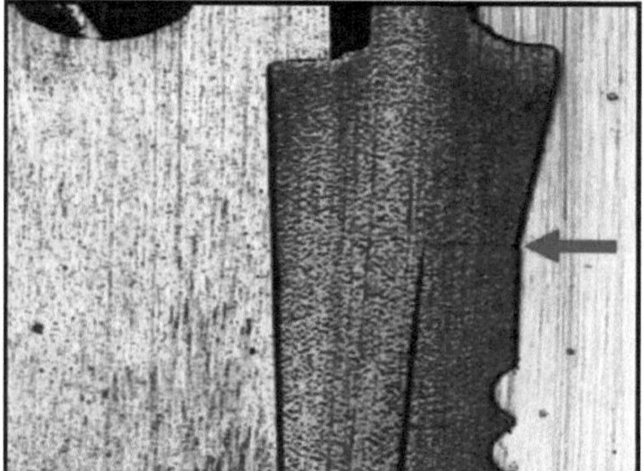

FIGURA 18   - Indexed internal hexagon connection (gap width at implant/abutment interface = 1.9µm. Optical microscope photograph (63 X).

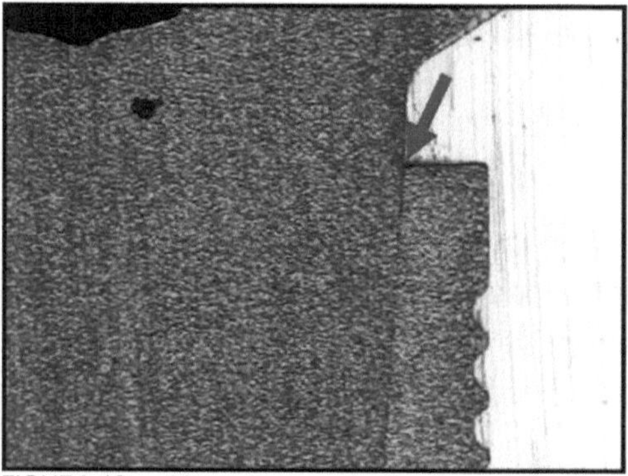

FIGURA 19   - Morse cone connection (gap width at implant/abutment interface = 0.4µm. Optical microscope photograph (63 X).

The results were analysed statistically using the multiple comparison of proportions test proposed by ZAR[7] (1999), executed via macro, provided by the Minitab for Windows statistical program, version 15, (www. minitab.com). Kaplan-Meier analysis was also carried out to compare the survival curves (probability of no infiltration up to 7 days) of the implant/prosthetic abutment combinations. The Log-Rank and Wilcoxon statistical methods were used to compare the probability distribution curves for the absence of infiltration.

CHAPTER 5

RESULTS

The study sample consisted of 50 samples of 3 models of prosthetic connections and their respective implants: Morse cone, external hexagon and indexed internal hexagon, for a total of 150 sets of abutments and implants.

Samples that showed immediate external contamination and those that showed neither turbidity nor viability within 7 days were discarded from the study. As a result, the number of samples considered for calculating the research results was reduced and is shown in Table 2:

Table 2: Number of samples discarded and considered in the study.

Group	Total samples	Samples discarded due to external contamination	Samples discarded as unviable after 7 days	Samples included
G1 (HE)	50	02	10	38
G2 (HII)	50	01	08	41
G3 (CM)	50	00	10	40

Of the total number of connections (119), 7.56% showed infiltration during the 7-day assessment period. In the external hexagon group (G1), 4 samples (10.53%) showed bacterial infiltration through the interface between the abutment and the implant, in the indexed internal hexagon group (G2), 2 (4.88%) and in the cone morse group (G3), infiltration occurred in 3 samples (7.5%). The first null hypothesis (H_0 -i) of this investigation was rejected (Tableai).

Table 1 - Number and percentage of samples with bacterial infiltration in different prophetic connections over a 7-day period.

Prosthetic connector	Number of samples with bacterial infiltration	Sample size (n)	% bacterial infiltration
HE	4	38	10,53
HII	2	41	4,88
CM	3	40	7,50

When the three proportions of infiltration were compared with each other, the statistical test recommended by Zar[7] (1999) showed that the second null hypothesis (H_{-02}) was accepted, i.e. the same prevalence of infiltration occurred between the three prosthetic connections.

The behaviour of the samples - in terms of infiltration as a function of time - was assessed using the Kaplan-Meier method (especially appropriate in studies involving a small number of samples).

The three survival curves for each of the connections are shown below.

In the external hexagon group (G1), the first infiltration occurred after 3 days of immersion. The second and third samples showed infiltration after 5 days and the fourth after 7 days (Figure 20).

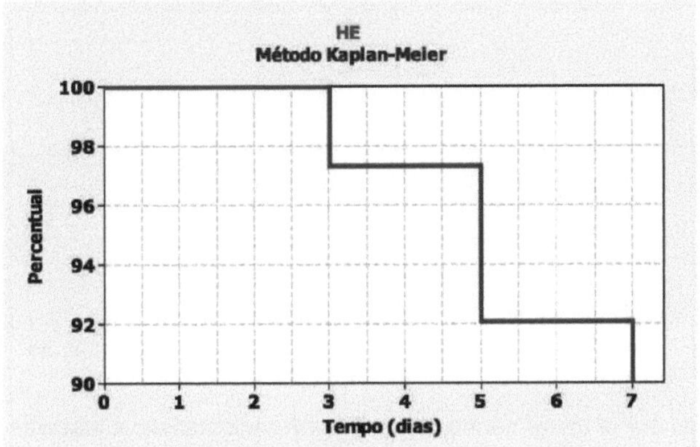

FIGURA 20   - Percentage probability estimated by the Kaplan-Meier method of external hexagon samples that did not infiltrate in relation to time (days).

In the HII group (G2), the first infiltration occurred after 5 days of immersion, followed by a second infiltration after 6 days of immersion (Figure 21).

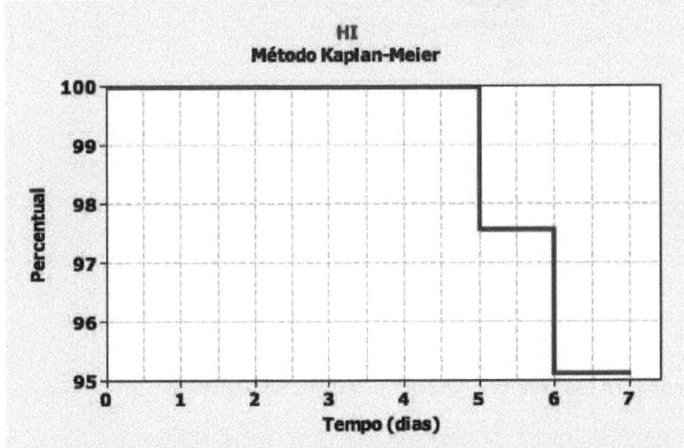

FIGURA 21   Percentage probability estimated by the Kaplan-Meier method of the indexed internal hexagon samples that did not infiltrate in relation to time (days).

Group CM (G3) showed the first infiltration after 2 days of immersion. On the third day, a second implant showed infiltration. And on the fourth day the third implant showed infiltration, with no further infiltration occurring for this type of connection until the end of the

7 days (Figure 22).

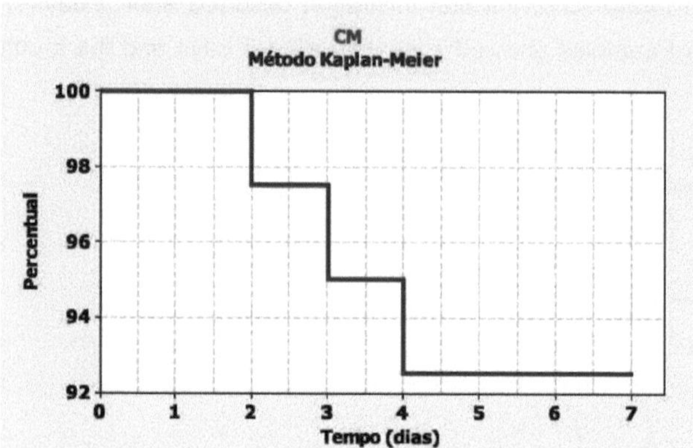

FIGURE 22: Percentage probability estimated by the Kaplan-Meier method of Morse cone samples that did not infiltrate in relation to time (days).

To better assess the behaviour of these connections, the log-rank statistical test was applied. It can be seen that the probability distribution curves of the different types of prophetic connections also did not differ from one another (x^2 = 0.879; gl = 2; p=0.644), indicating that the three connections showed a similar behaviour in terms of infiltration in relation to the time elapsed, which can be seen in Figure 23.

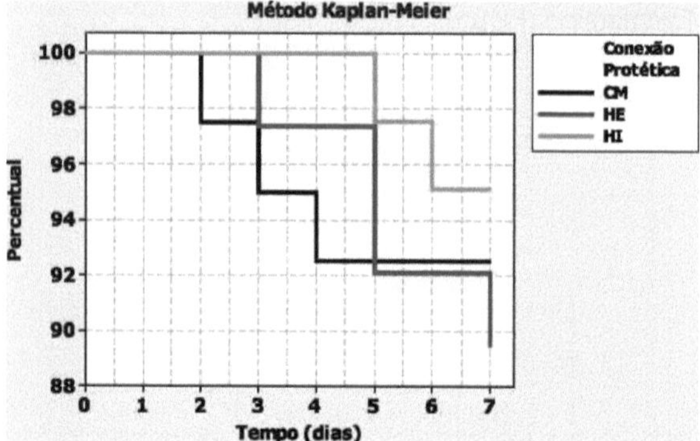

FIGURE 23 - Comparison of the survival curve of the different types of prophetic connections.

CHAPTER 6

DISCUSSION

The current literature and that of recent years has been increasingly concerned with studying the possible causes of implant treatment failure. Despite the excellent success rates in rehabilitations with osseointegrated implants, failures have been described and related to surgical techniques, mechanical and microbiological factors, often acting in association[14,36,41] . In the long term, the role of microorganisms must be considered in implant survival. Bacteria and their by-products can cause inflammatory reactions in the peri-implant soft tissues .[12,28,35,44]

Three types of prosthetic connections, widely used by professionals in the field, were evaluated in this study: external hexagon (EH), indexed internal hexagon (IHE) and Morse cone (MMC). The quality of the adaptation of the interface between the abutment and the implant was assessed by analysing bacterial infiltration. The three types showed low rates of bacterial infiltration, with no significant difference between them. The first null hypothesis H_{0-1} was rejected and the second (H0-2) was accepted.

Bacterial infiltration through the interface between the abutment and the implant can basically be assessed in two ways: by checking whether bacteria pass into the implant[5,17,26,29,36,37,40,50] or in the opposite direction[3,15,16,17,19,26,29,46,47,50] . Bacterial infiltration from the external environment into the implant better represents the *in vivo* situation, but for *in vitro* tests, this situation can present certain disadvantages and problems. The abutments are connected to the implants under sterile conditions, immersed in a bacterial suspension, and infiltration through the interface between the abutment and the implant has to be proven by the presence of bacteria on the inside of the implant. Therefore, due to the need to disconnect the assembly for verification, the sample can only be evaluated once after a certain period, preventing a longitudinal evaluation.

The methodology used in this research was determined on the basis of meticulous pilot studies. One of them showed that verifying the passage of bacteria into the implant can make the results unreliable, because in order to verify whether there has been bacterial infiltration, it is necessary to carry out external disinfection before separating the abutment and implant. Due to the difficulty in previously sealing the interface between the abutment and the implant, this procedure can take the disinfectant agent inside the implant, i.e. via the same route of bacterial penetration, masking the results.

In the study by Besimo *et al.*[5] , 1999, which analysed bacterial infiltration into the implants, no sample showed infiltration. The authors related the results to the use of a chlorhexidine-based varnish, but disinfection was carried out before the abutments were opened for analysis, which may not have guaranteed the viability of the bacteria. The same occurred in the study by Dibart *et aú*[7] , 2005, in which, after external disinfection to observe the inside of the implants, no infiltration was observed in any sample.

Checking the passage of bacteria in the opposite direction, i.e. from inside the implant to the external environment, seems to be more reliable, but external contamination can occur due to microorganisms leaking out after inoculation and installation of the abutment[3,15,19,29,47] . In 2008, Faria *et aP* carried out a research study, used as a pilot study for the present investigation, in which two methodologies were compared, verifying external contamination after inoculation and torque in three types of prosthetic connections: external hexagon (HE), indexed internal hexagon (HII) and cone morse (CM). Twenty samples of each type of connection were used. In methodology 1, 0.7 pl of *Escherichia coli* suspension was inoculated inside the implants and the respective abutments connected with a torque of 20Ncm. In Method 2, an *E. coli colony* was inoculated into the apical portion of the abutment screw before the torque was applied. The assemblies were deposited and rolled onto plates with TSA (tryptic soy agar, Himedia) and covered with liquid TSA. After rolling, the plates were taken to a bacteriological oven at 37^e C to check for colony growth after 24 hours. In methodology 1, the percentage of external contamination was 5, 60 and 45 per cent for HE, HII and CM, respectively. In methodology 2, it was 10, 5 and 0 per cent for HE, HII and CM, respectively. In this pilot study, it was concluded that the bacterial colony inoculation methodology showed less external contamination during the experiment for the HII and CM groups, resulting in fewer samples being discarded and greater efficiency in data collection. As for the samples from the HE group, there were no statistical differences between the two methodologies.

Jansen *et al.*[29] , 1997, used the methodology of inoculating an *E.coli* suspension inside the implant to evaluate 13 implant systems, with different types of prosthetic connections, and noted the problem of an excessive number of samples with immediate external contamination in the conical connection systems. More than 50 per cent of the samples were discarded for this reason (Ankylos Degussa/Dentsply: out of 37 samples, 21 with external contamination; Astra - Astra Tech: out of 40 samples, 24 with external contamination). In the case of the external hexagon connection, the rate was lower, with the problem occurring in 8 of the 25 samples from the Branemark - Nobel Biocare system. The other systems with different types of internal connections studied by the authors had lower numbers, ranging from 0 to 5 samples discarded due to external contamination. In the study by Guindy *et al.*[26] , 1998, in 30 samples of internal hexagon connections (Ha-Ti, Mathys

Dental Implants), inoculated with 2pl of *staphylococcus aureus* suspension, there was no external contamination. All showed infiltration. Unlike the method used to check for external contamination in our study and those of other authors[29,47] , they carried out the test with paper cones rolled over the external portion of the interface, which may not have been efficient in assessing the occurrence of suspension leakage contaminating the external environment.

The same internal hexagon implant system (Ha-Ti, Mathys Dental Implants) from the study by Guindy *et al.*[26] , 1998, was evaluated in the study by Besimo *et al.*[5] , 1999, but with the use of a chlorhexidine varnish on the interfaces. The opposite results were found, with none of the samples showing infiltration. The varnish may have prevented bacteria from penetrating, but disinfection was carried out with 70% alcohol after inoculating a 2pl suspension of *Staphylococcus aureus* prior to introducing the set in sterile solution. Furthermore, they did not observe the viability of the bacteria after a total observation period of 7 days. The methodology applied may not lend credibility to the results.

In another pilot study, the viability time of the bacteria *(E.coli) was* also tested under the conditions proposed for this work. The maximum time in which the viability of the bacteria was observed was 7 days.

Based on the pilot studies carried out and the fact that bacterial penetration can occur in both directions[50] , in our research we opted for the reverse technique by inoculating a colony of bacteria inside the implant, with an evaluation period of 7 days. As a result, the number of samples with immediate external contamination was very low: one in group 1 (external hexagon), two in group 2 (indexed internal hexagon) and none in group 3 (Morse cone). On the other hand, in order to validate the results, a bacterial viability test was carried out on all the samples that did not show infiltration after 7 days. Those that did not show viability were excluded from the study, which resulted in approximately 20% of samples being discarded in each group (see Appendix).

We consider it extremely important to assess the viability of the bacteria at the end of the experiment, as it is unwise to state that there was no infiltration without this confirmation. In most of the studies we consulted ' ' '3515,16,171929 "46 there were samples without bacterial infiltration, but none of these authors bothered to check the viability of the bacteria previously inoculated into the implants, thus jeopardising the reliability of the results. A more dubious scientific situation occurs in the studies that presented a 0% infiltration rate for some prosthetic connection systems (Besimo *et al.*[5] , 1999 - HA-TI system, Mathys Dental Implants; Dibart *et al.*[7] , 2005 - Bicon Dental implants system; Santana[46] , 2007 - Titamax cone morse, Neodent and Ankylos systems, Dentsply Friadent).

Escherichia coli is a Gram-negative bacterium. It takes the form of a bacillus, measuring 1.1 to 1.5 μm in diameter and 2 to 6 μm in length. It was chosen for this study because it has motility and is widely used in *in vitro* studies to study sterilisation, disinfection and contamination[16,29,47]. It is also easy to handle in the laboratory, multiplies in a short time (20 min) and can be found in the oral cavity of healthy individuals.

Jansen *etal.*[29], 1997, evaluated bacterial infiltration in 13 types of prosthetic connections, including external hexagon, internal hexagon and Morse cone. They found bacterial infiltration in all types of connections. The results of the present study are not in agreement with those obtained by the authors who stated that the good adaptation between abutments and implants, observed in Scanning Electron Microscopy (SEM) images, is not capable of preventing bacterial infiltration. Comparisons can be made between some of the systems evaluated by Jansen *et al.* and those in this study. In the conical connection samples, the infiltration rate was 50% for the Ankylos - Dentsply Friadent system (n=16), 69% for the Astra - Astra Tech system (n=16) and 96% for the ITI Bonefit - Straumann system (n=23), results that are quite different from those obtained in our study, in which, of the 40 cone morse connection samples, only 3 showed bacterial infiltration, representing a percentage of 7.5%. The same can be seen when comparing the results of the external hexagon connections, with 82% infiltration in the Branemark - Nobel Biocare system (n=17), compared to 10.53% (n=38) in the Conexão system. The other internal connections of different configurations also showed high infiltration rates, ranging from 38 to 100 per cent, contrary to the data obtained from the indexed internal hexagon connection with only 4.88 per cent infiltration (n=41). The higher percentage rate observed by the authors is not related to the longer assessment period (14 days) compared to the present study (7 days), as the total number of infiltrated samples had already occurred on the seventh day of observation. The unfavourable result obtained may be related to the fact that the torque procedure for adapting the abutments was not carried out. We disagree with the justification given by the authors who report that this procedure is not commonly carried out by clinicians due to the need for repeated removal and insertion of the abutments for various reasons.

The importance of the ideal torque used on the screw that retains the prosthetic connector must be taken into account, as it can affect the size of the micro-space at the interface between the abutment and the implant[25,53]. In a study of dye infiltration at the interface between the abutment and the implant of five implant systems available on the market, varying the torque (10, 20 Nem and that recommended by the manufacturer), Gross *et al.*[25] (1999) observed that microleakage decreased significantly with increasing torque in all systems. The authors suggested that bacterial by-products and nutrients necessary for bacterial growth may also pass through this space, contributing to the bad odour and peri-implant diseases observed clinically.

The occurrence of bacterial infiltration through the interface between the abutment and the implant is presumed to be due to many factors, such as the precision of the fit between the components, the degree of micro-movement between the components[47] and the torque forces used to connect them[25].

It can be considered that the biological characteristics related to successful rehabilitation with implants are closely related to the mechanical characteristics of the prosthetic components involved. In this study, a small number of samples showed infiltration through the interface between the abutment and the implant. The torque indicated by the manufacturer was applied and the optical microscopy images showed adequate adaptation of the connections, but the test was carried out without the application of loads that would simulate the clinical situation of chewing. This may explain the low incidence of bacterial infiltration observed in our study, compared to the higher amount observed *in* some *in v/o* studies[13,38,42,45]. The stability of the prosthetic connections in the face of the masticatory loads received may have influenced the adaptation between the components, opening cracks and allowing bacteria to penetrate. Binon[6], in 1996, showed that there is a direct correlation between hexagon maladaptation and prosthetic abutment screw loss. According to the author, the greater the rotational freedom, the greater the likelihood of the abutment screw coming loose.

The dynamic behaviour of prosthetic connections on implants when faced with the possibility of bacterial infiltration was studied by Steinebrunner *et al.*[47], 2005. The authors proposed a new *in vitro* study model to assess bacterial infiltration at the interfaces between abutments and implants, applying dynamic forces in a chewing simulator. They evaluated external hexagon connection systems, internal connections and cone morse. Unlike our results, in which the percentage infiltration rate for external hexagon, indexed and cone morse was 10.53%, 4.88% and 7.5% respectively, the authors obtained 100% infiltration in the 5 implant systems evaluated. However, the number of cycles required before infiltration occurred varied between the systems. The average number of chewing cycles required for *E.coli to infiltrate* the interfaces was: 24,300 for Screw-Vent - Zimmer Dental (mixed connection - internal hexagon and Morse cone); 43,200 for Frialit-2 hermetic system - Dentsply Friadent (internal hexagon with silicone sealing cylinder); 64.800 for Replace - Nobel Biocare (internal tube-in-tube connection with fixation guides); 172,800 for Branemark - Nobel Biocare (external hexagon); and 345,600 for Camlog - Altatech (internal tube-in-tube connection with fixation guides). The authors considered the connections that obtained the best results to be more stable, because they minimised micro-movement in the face of the loads received. The torque may be related to these results, as the external hexagon system, in which the recommended torque was 45 Nem, obtained a higher average number of cycles until infiltration occurred, compared to the internal connection systems, with torques ranging from 20 to 35 Nem. In the present study, the torque applied was 20 Nem for the three types of connections, as recommended by the manufacturer, and the external hexagon connections had a higher infiltration rate than the internal ones. On the other hand, in the study by Steinebrunner et al.[47], 2005, the mixed connection system (internal hexagon and Morse cone) showed the worst results, with the lowest average number of cycles, which may indicate that the combination of connections is not as efficient in promoting stability of the set. Although not statistically different, we also obtained better results with the indexed internal hexagon connection (4.88%) compared to the Morse cone (7.50%). We believe that a greater torque force could be indicated for the Morse cone, thus increasing the stability promoted by friction between the conical walls of the abutment and implant.

The stability of cone morse and indexed internal hexagon prosthetic connections was assessed by Faria et al.[24] in 2008. The tests were carried out by assessing the torque force required to disconnect the abutment from its respective implant after mechanical cycling fatigue. In this study, the Morse cone connection obtained the best results, proving to be more stable in the face of the forces applied. In a finite element study, Merz et al.[32], 2000, showed the different mechanical principles of function of external hexagon and Morse cone connections. The forces applied at different angles highlighted the importance of the conical connection in reducing the load transmitted to the screw portion of the abutment, preventing it from loosening. In addition, while the tension is compensated, the conical friction guarantees anti-rotational stability between the implant and the abutment. It can be considered that the mechanical stability of the Morse cone connection combined with the excellent quality of the interface against bacterial infiltration, as shown in this study, makes this type of connection a good option for rehabilitations with osseointegrated implants.

Dibart et al.[7], 2005, observed a gap of less than 0.5µm in the interface between the abutment and the implant in a Morse cone connection, considering this space insufficient for the passage of bacteria. They analysed bacterial infiltration from the external to the internal environment of the implant. The results showed no bacteria inside the implants after SEM analysis, in an evaluation period of just 24 hours. They also carried out infiltration in the opposite direction, from the inside of the implant to the outside, at 24, 48 and 72 hours. Of the 20 samples tested (10 for each type of test), none showed bacterial infiltration through the interface between the abutment and the implant. The authors related the favourable result to the quality of the adaptation provided by the Morse cone connection system. Although the results are in agreement with those of the present study, we consider the evaluation period proposed by the authors to be insufficient, based on the fact that we observed turbidity of the medium in some samples after 72 hours. In addition, in the test to verify the passage of bacteria from the internal to the external environment, the viability of the bacteria inside the implant was not assessed, as was done in the present study.

Most prosthetic components for implants are made up of two parts: an abutment and a retaining screw. There are also solid abutments that are threaded into the implants and do not require screws for retention. In our research, as well as *in* other studies *in* v/tro[5,29,40] [47], it was considered that two-part abutments, because they have two routes of penetration for bacteria (the interface between the abutment and the implant and the abutment screw hole), should be kept partially immersed, keeping only the interface region in contact with the sterile solution. This care was not taken by other authors[3,15] [16,19] [46] who completely submerged all their samples, preventing the real infiltration from being seen only at the interface between the abutment and the implant. In their study, Quirynem *et al.[40]* (1994) observed low contamination in partially submerged abutment and implant assemblies compared to fully submerged ones. Some authors have sealed prior to immersion with guttapercha and cyanocrylate[16,19], but the efficiency of this procedure has not been tested.

External hexagon connections from the Conexão Sitemas de Prótese system, among others, were tested in the studies by Cravinhos[15], 2003, Amaral[3], 2003, and Dias[16], 2007. Methodologies similar to ours, but without the same precautions mentioned above, were used and the results were quite discrepant, reaching percentage rates of samples with infiltration of 71.43%[15], 90%[3] and 62.5%[16], compared to the rate of 10.5% for the external hexagon group, reached in our research. This discrepancy may be related to the total immersion of the samples, keeping the two routes of bacterial penetration in contact with the sterile environment.

The clinical phenomenon of bleeding and bad odour characteristic of anaerobic bacteria that occurs when removing abutments and healers may be the result of the effects of bacterial micro-infiltration. Efforts have been made by manufacturers to improve the quality of this interface.

Three different types of prosthetic connections from the same manufacturer were tested and showed similar behaviour with regard to bacterial infiltration. Other manufacturers produce components with connections that are compatible with each other, with the same configuration, especially the pioneering external hexagon connection. In the study by Gross *et al.[25]*, 1999, of the 5 systems evaluated in the study, 3 were external hexagon (Spline - Sulzer Calcitek (*Spliney* connection, CeraOne - Nobel Biocare (external hexagon); Steri-oss - Steri-oss (external hexagon); 3i - Implant Inovation (external hexagon); ITI - Straumann (cone morse). They used a solution of gentian violet diluted in distilled water, introduced under pressure, to assess the sealing of the interfaces at different torques (10Ncm, 20Ncm and the manufacturer's recommendation). All infiltrated, but the amount varied between systems and torques, with significantly less infiltration with the recommended torque. The Morse cone system (ITI) showed a higher average infiltration rate than the external hexagon system, a result that is not in line with the findings of this study. Although the methodologies are different, a certain comparison can be made between the results of Gross *et al.*[25] , 1999, and those of the present study, in which the behaviour of the interfaces to the passage of bacteria was observed in approximately 40 samples of each type of connection for 7 days, simulating *in vitro, in a* reverse manner, what would happen *in vivo.* In the work by Gross *et al.*[25] , 1999, only three samples of each system were used in which a low molecular weight dye diluted in distilled water was introduced under pressure to assess its passage through the interfaces, observed at three time intervals (5, 20 and 80 minutes). The small number of samples used by the authors may have been insufficient to guarantee the results. On the other hand, it should be borne in mind that the three systems with the same interface configuration (external hexagon) had different behaviour. It can be inferred that the quality of the interface between the abutment and the implant is directly related to the manufacturing system and may vary between the same types of connection configurations.

Various implant systems produce conical Morse-type prosthetic connections. Merz *et al.*[32] , 2000, showed in their finite element study the mechanical advantages of the system, but the literature indicates that the quality of this adaptation can vary between different manufacturers. Santana[46] , in 2007, obtained different responses regarding the percentage of bacterial infiltration through the interfaces of 5 cone morse systems in 14 days of evaluation: AR morse, Conexão Sistemas de Prostostosthética - 20%; Titamax cone morse, Neodent - 0%; Titanium Fix cone morse, AS Tech -100%; Straumann, Straumann AG - 100%; and Ankylos, Dentsply Friadent - 0%).

A wide variety of microorganisms seem to be able to infiltrate the interface between the abutment and the implant. Some species identified as *Actinobacillus actinomycetemcomitans, Porphyromonas gingivallis, Campylobacter rectus, Bacteroides spp., Fusobacterium spp. and Peptostreptococcus micros,* have been associated with peri-implantitis[33 , 3943,51] . These microorganisms are considered small compared to the cracks found at the interfaces between abutments and implants.

The aim of this study was to assess the behaviour of different types of prosthetic connections in relation to the possibility of bacterial infiltration. Components from the same manufacturer were used, which standardised the production quality of the material. Based on the literature review, we believe that the quality of the adaptation of the interface between abutments and implants, as well as the stability of the prosthetic connections of the various existing implant systems, may be directly related to the different results found in the various studies.

CHAPTER 7

CONCLUSIONS

In view of the results found in the study, it was concluded that:

a) *in vitro* bacterial contamination through the interfaces between abutments and implants occurred to a small extent in all groups;

b) bacterial infiltration occurred similarly in the three types of prophetic connections evaluated, despite the different interface configurations between the abutments and implants.

REFERENCES*

1 . Abrahamsson I, Berglundh T, Moon IS, Lindhe J. Peri-implant tissues at submerged and non-submerged titanium implants. J Clin PeriodontoL 1999 Sep;26(9):600-7.

2 . Adell R, Lekholm U, Rockler B, Brànemark PI. A 15-year study of osseointegrated implants in the treatment of the edentulous jaw. Int J Oral Surg. 1981 Dec;10(6):387-416.

3 . Amaral JIQ. In vitro analysis of bacterial infiltration and maladaptations at the implant/prosthetic connector interface in five endosseous implant systems [thesis]. Piracicaba: Piracicaba School of Dentistry: State University of Campinas; 2003.

4 . Avivi-Arber L, Zarb GA. Clinicai effectiveness of implant-supported single-tooth replacement: the Toronto Study. Int J Oral Maxillofac Implants. 1996 May-Jun;11(3):311-21.

5 . Besimo CE, Guindy JS, Lewetag D, Meyer J. Prevention of bacterial leakage into and from prefabricated screw-retained crowns on implants in vitro. Int J Oral Maxillofac Implants, 1999 Sep- Oct;14(5):654-60.

6 . Binon PP. The effect of implant/abutment hexagonal misfit on screw joint stability. Int J Prosthodont.1996 Mar-Apr;9(2):149-60.

7 . Jerrold ZAR. Biostatistical Analysis. 4th Ed. 1999.

---

* Based on:

International Committee of Medical Journal Editors. Bibliographic Services Division. Uniform requirements for manuscripts submitted to biomedical journals: simple referents [homepage on the Internet]. Bethesda: US National Library; c2003 [available 2006 Feb; cited 20 Mar]. Available at : http://www.nilm.nih.gov/bsd/uniform_requeriments.html

8 . Block MS, Kent JN. Long-term follow-up on hydroxylapatite-coated cylindrical dental implants: a comparison between developmental and recent periods.J Oral Maxillofac Surg. 1994 Sep;52(9):937-43.

9 . Brânemark PI. Osseointegration and its experimental background. J Prosthet Dent. 1983 Sep;50(3):399-410.

10 . Brânemark PI, Adell R, Breine U, Hansson BO, Lindstrom J, *et al...* Intra-osseous anchorage of dental prostheses. I. Experimental studies. Scand J Plast Reconstr Surg. 1969;3(2):81-100.

11 . Brânemark PI, Zarb GA, Albresktsson, T.A. Tissue-integrated prostheses: osseointegration in clinical dentistry. Chicago: Quintessence, 1987. 350p.

12 Broggini N, McManus LM, Hermann JS, Medina RU, Oates TW, *et al...* Persistent acute inflammation at the implant-abutment interface. J Dent Res. 2003 Mar.;82(3):232-7.

13 Callan DP, Cobb CM, Williams KB. DNA probe identification of bacteria colonising internal surfaces of the implant-abutment interface: a preliminary study. J Periodontol. 2005 Jan;76(1):115- 20.

14 Covani U, Marconcini S, Crespi R, Barone A. Bacterial plaque colonisation around dental implant surfaces. Implant Dent. 2006 Sep;15(3):298-304.

15 Cravinhos JCP. In vitro analysis of bacterial contamination at the implant/prosthetic connector interface in three endosseous implant systems [dissertation]. Piracicaba: Piracicaba School of Dentistry, State University of Campinas; 2003.

16 . Dias ECLCM. Descriptive analysis of the degree of adaptation of prosthetic abutments to osseointegrated implants and their effect on bacterial infiltration: an in vitro study [dissertation]. Duque de Caxias: Unigranrio University; 2007.

17 . Dibart S, Warbington M, Su MF, Skobe Z. In vitro evaluation of the implant-abutment bacterial seal: the locking taper system. Int J Oral Maxillofac Implants. 2005 Sep-Oct;20(5):732-7.

18 Ding TA, Woody RD, Higginbottom FL, Miller BH. Evaluation of the ITI Morse taper implant/abutment design with an internai modification. Int J Oral Maxillofac Implants. 2003 Nov- Dec;18(6):865-72.

19 .do Nascimento C, Barbosa RE, Issa JP, Watanabe E, Ito IY, *et al.* Bacterial leakage along the implant-abutment interface of premachined or cast components. Int J Oral Maxillofac Surg. 2008 Feb;37(2):177-80.

20 Ekfeldt A, Carlsson GE, Borjesson G. Clinicai evaluation of single-tooth restorations supported by osseointegrated implants: a retrospective study. Int J Oral Maxillofac

Implants. 1994 Mar-Apr; 9(2):179-83.

21 Esposito M, Hirsch JM, Lekholm U, Thomsen P. Biological factors contributing to failures of osseointegrated oral implants (I). Success criteria and epidemiology. Eur J Oral Sei. 1998 Feb;106(1): 527-51.

22 Esposito M, Hirsch JM, Lekholm U, Thomsen P. Biological factors contributing to failures of osseointegrated oral implants. (II). Etiopathogenesis. Eur J Oral Sei. 1998 Jun;106(3):721-64.

23 . Faria R, May LG, Paschotto DR, Oliveira LD, Jorge AOC, Bottino MA. Comparative study between two methodologies for assessing bacterial infiltration at the implant-abutment interface. Proceedings of the 2nd Annual Meeting of the Brazilian Prosthesis and Implant Recycling Group; 2008. Campos do Jordão: Brazilian Prosthesis and Implant Recycling Group; 2008.

24 . Faria R, Zamboni SC, Goiatá F, Castro H, Barca DC, Bottino MA. Removal torque of taper and indexed abutment: mechanical loading effect. In Press 2008.

25 . Gross M, Abramovich I, Weiss EL Microleakage at the abutment- implant interface of osseointegrated implants: a comparative study. Int J Oral Maxillofac Implants 1999 Jan-Feb;14(1):94-100.

26 Guindy JS, Besimo CE, Besimo R, Schiel H, Meyer J. Bacterial leakage into and from prefabricated screw-retained implant-borne crowns in vitro. J Oral Rehabil. 1998 Jun;25(6):403-8.

27 Henry PJ, Tolman DE, Bolender C. The applicability of osseointegrated implants in the treatment of partially edentulous patients: three-year results of a prospective multicentre study. Quintessence Int. 1993 Feb;24(2):123-9.

28 Hermann JS, Schoolfield JD, Schenk RK, Buser D, Cochran DL. Influence of the size of the microgap on crestai bone changes around titanium implants. A histometric evaluation of unloaded non- submerged implants in the canine mandible. J Periodontol. 2001 Oct;72(10): 1372-83.

29 Jansen VK, Conrads G, Richter EJ. Microbial leakage and marginal fit of the implant-abutment interface. Int J Oral Maxillofac Implants. 1997 Jul-Aug;12(4):527-40.

30 King GN, Hermann JS, Schoolfield JD, Buser D, Cochran DL. Influence of the size of the microgap on crestai bone levels in non- submerged dental implants: a radiographic study in the canine mandible. J Periodontol. 2002 Oct;73(10):1111 -7.

31 Leonhardt A, Grondahl K, Bergstrom C, Lekholm U. Long-term follow-up of osseointegrated titanium implants using clinical, radiographic and microbiological parameters. Clin Oral Implants Res. 2002 Apr;13(2):127-32.

32 . Merz BR, Hunenbart S, Belser UC. Mechanics of the implant- abutment connection: an 8-degree taper compared to a butt joint connection. Int J Oral Maxillofac Implants 2000 Jul-Aug;15(4):519- 26.

33 Mombelli A, Lang NP. Microbial aspects of implant dentistry. Periodontol 2000.1994 Feb;4:74-80.

34 . Norton MR. Multiple single-tooth implant restorations in the posterior jaws: maintenance of marginal bone levels with reference to the implant-abutment microgap. Int J Oral Maxillofac Implants. 2006 Sep-Oct;21(5):777-84.

35 .0'Mahony A, MacNeill SR, Cobb CM. Design features that may influence bacterial plaque retention: a retrospective analysis of failed implants. Quintessence Int. 2000 Apr;31(4):249-56.

36 . Piattelli A, Scarano A, Paolantonio M, Assenza B, Leghissa GC, et al. Fluids and microbial penetration in the internal part of cement- retained versus screw-retained implant-abutment connections. J Periodontol 2001 Sep;72(9):1146-50.

37 . Piattelli A, Vrespa G, Petrone G, Iezzi G, Annibali S, Scarano A. Role of the microgap between implant and abutment: a retrospective histologic evaluation in monkeys. J Periodontol. 2003 Mar;74(3):346-52.

38 Persson LG, Lekholm U, Leonhardt A, Dahlén G, Lindhe J. Bacterial colonisation on internai surfaces of Brânemark system implant components. Clin Oral Implants Res. 1996 Jun;7(2):90-5.

39 . Pongnarisom NJ, Gemmell E, Tan AE, Henry PJ, Marshall RI, etal. Inflammation associated with implants with different surface types. Clin Oral Implants Res. 2007 Feb;18(1):114-25.

40 Quirynen M, Bollen CM, Eyssen H, van Steenberghe D. Microbial penetration along the implant components of the Brânemark system. An in vitro study. Clin Oral Implants Res. 1994 Dec;5(4):239-44.

41 Quirynen M, de Soete M, van Steenberghe D. Infections risks for oral implants: a review of the literature. Clin Oral Implants Res 2002 Feb,13(1):1-19.

42 . Quirynen M, van Steenberghe D. Bacterial colonisation of the internai part of two-stage implants. An in vivo study. Clin Oral Implants Res. 1993 Sep;4(3):158-61.

43 . Quirynen M, Vogels R, Peeters W, van Steenberghe D, Naert I, Haffajee A. Dynamics of initial subgingival colonisation of 'pristine' peri-implant pockets. Clin Oral Implants Res. 2006 Feb, 17(1): 25- 37.

44-Ricci G, Aimetti M, Stablum W, Guasti A. Crestai bone resorption 5 years after implant loading: clinicai and radiologic results with a 2- stage implant system. Int J Oral

Maxillofac Implants. 2004 Jul-Aug;19(4):597-602.

45 Rimondini L, Marin C, Brunella F, Fini M. Internal contamination of a 2-component implant system after occlusal loading and provisionally luted reconstruction with or without a washer device. J PeriodontoL 2001 Dec;72(12):1652-7.

46 . Santana WM. Evaluation of microbiological infiltration of the implant-abutment interface in internal hexagon and conemorse connections of osseointegrated implants [dissertation]. Goiânia: Federal University of Goiás School of Dentistry, 2007.

47 Steinebrunner L, Wolfart S, Bossmann K, Kern M. In vitro evaluation of bacterial leakage along the implant-abutment interface of different implant Systems. Int J Oral Maxillofac Implants. 2005 Nov-Dec;20(6):875-81.

48 Tarnow DP, Magner AW, Fletcher P. The effect of the distance from the contact point to the crest of bone on the presence or absence of the interproximal dental papilla. J PeriodontoL 1992 Dec;63(12):995-6.

49 Todescan FF, Pustiglioni FE, Imbronito AV, Albrektsson T, Gioso M. Influence of the microgap in the peri-implant hard and soft tissues: a histomorphometric study in dogs. Int J Oral Maxillofac Implants. 2002 Jul-Aug;17(4):467-72.

50 Traversy MC, Birek P. Fluid and microbial leakage of implant- abutment assembly *in vitro.* [J Dent Res 1992;71(754): 1909.

51 .van Winkelhoff AJ, Goene RJ, Benschop C, Folmer T. Early colonisation of dental implants by putative periodontal pathogens in partially edentulous patients. Clin Oral Implants Res. 2000 Dec;11(6):511-20.

52 Weber HP, Crohin CC, Fiorellini JP. A 5-year prospective clinical and radiographic study of non-submerged dental implants. Clin Oral Implants Res. 2000 Apr;11(2): 144-53.

53 Weiss EI, Kozak D, Gross MD. Effect of repeated closures on opening torque values in seven abutment-implant systems. J Prosthet Dent. 2000 Aug;84(2): 194-9.

54 . Zarb GA, Schmitt A. The longitudinal clinical effectiveness of osseointegrated dental implants in posterior partially edentulous patients. Int J Prosthodont. 1993 Mar-Apr;6(2): 189-96.

APPENDIX A: Data related to the external hexagon samples (G1)

	Connection	Immediate external contamination (EC)	Turbidity (T)	Viability (V)
1.	HE		-	V - DISCONTINUED
2.	HE	CE - DISCARDED	CE - DISCARDED	CE - DISCARDED
3.	HE		-	+
4.	HE			V - DISCONTINUED
5.	HE		-	+
6.	HE		-	+
7.	HE		-	+
8.	HE		-	+
9.	HE		-	V - DISCONTINUED

			Turbidity (T)	Viability (V)
10.	HE		T-FREE	T-FREE
11.	HE		-	+
12.	HE		-	+
13.	HE		-	+
14.	HE		-	+
15.	HE		-	+
16.	HE		-	+
17.	HE	CE - DISCARDED	CE - DISCARDED	CE - DISCARDED
18.	HE		-	V-FREE
19.	HE		-	+
20.	HE		-	+
21.	HE		T-FREE	T-FREE
22.	HE		-	+
23.	HE		-	+
24.	HE		-	V - DISCONTINUED
25.	HE		-	V-FREE
26.	HE		-	+
27.	HE		-	+
28.	HE		-	+
29.	HE		-	+
30.	HE		-	+
31.	HE		-	+
32.	HE		-	+
33.	HE		-	+
34.	HE		-	+
35.	HE		-	V - DISCONTINUED
36.	HE		-	+
37.	HE		-	V - DISCONTINUED
38.	HE		-	+
39.	HE		-	+
40.	HE		-	+
41.	HE		-	+
42.	HE		T- DISCONTINUED	T-FREE
43.	HE		-	+
44.	HE		-	+
45.	HE		-	+
46.	HE		-	+
47.	HE		T-FREE	T-FREE
48.	HE		-	+
49.	HE		-	V-FREE
50.	HE		-	V - DISCONTINUED

APPENDIX B: Data related to the indexed internal hexagon samples (G2)

	Connection	Immediate external contamination (EC)	Turbidity (T)	Viability (V)
51.	HII		-	+
52.	HII		-	V - DISCONTINUED
53.	HII		-	+
54.	HII		-	V - DISCONTINUED
55.	HII		-	+
56.	HII		-	+
57.	HII		-	+
58.	HII		-	+
59.	HII	CE - DISCARDED	CE - DISCARDED	CE - DISCARDED
60.	HII		-	+
61.	HII		-	+
62.	HII		-	+
63.	HII		-	V - DISCONTINUED
64.	HII		-	+
65.	HII		-	+
66.	HII		-	+
67.	HII		-	+
68.	HII		-	+
69.	HII		-	+
70.	HII		-	V-FREE
71.	HII		-	V - DISCONTINUED
72.	HII		-	+
73.	HII		-	+
74.	HII		-	+
75.	HII		-	+
76.	HII		-	+
77.	HII		-	+

			-	+
78.	HII		-	+
79.	HII		-	+
80.	HII		-	V - DISCONTINUED
81.	HII		-	+
82.	HII		-	+
83.	HII		-	+
84.	HII		T- DISCONTINUED	T-FREE
85.	HII		-	+
86.	HII		-	+
87.	HII		-	V - DISCONTINUED
88.	HII		-	+
89.	HII		-	+
90.	HII		-	+
91.	HII		T-FREE	T-FREE
92.	HII		-	+
93.	HII		-	+
94.	HII		-	+
95.	HII		-	+
96.	HII		-	+
97.	HII		-	V - DISCONTINUED
98.	HII		-	+
99.	HII		-	+
100.	HII		-	+

APPENDIX C: Data related to morse cone samples (G3)

	Connection	Immediate external contamination (EC)	Turbidity (T)	Viability (V)
101.	CM		-	+
102.	CM		-	+
103.	CM		-	+
104.	CM		T- DISCONTINUED	T - DISCONTINUED
105.	CM		-	+
106.	CM		-	+
107.	CM		-	V-FREE
108.	CM		-	+
109.	CM		-	V - DISCONTINUED
110.	CM			V - DISCONTINUED
111.	CM		T- DISCONTINUED	T- DISCONTINUED
112.	CM			V - DISCONTINUED
113.	CM		-	+
114.	CM		-	V - DISCONTINUED
115.	CM		-	+
116.	CM		-	+
117.	CM			V - DISCONTINUED
118.	CM		-	V - DISCONTINUED
119.	CM		-	+
120.	CM		-	+
121.	CM		-	+
122.	CM		-	+
123.	CM		-	V - DISCONTINUED
124.	CM			V - DISCONTINUED
125.	CM		-	V - DISCONTINUED
126.	CM		-	+
127.	CM		-	+
128.	CM		-	+
129.	CM		-	+
130.	CM		-	V - DISCONTINUED
131.	CM		-	+
132.	CM		-	V - DISCONTINUED
133.	CM		-	+
134.	CM		-	+
135.	CM		-	+
136.	CM		-	+
137.	CM		T- DISCONTINUED	T- DISCONTINUED
138.	CM		-	+
139.	CM		-	+
140.	CM		-	+
141.	CM		-	+
142.	CM		-	+
143.	CM		-	+
144.	CM		-	+

145.	**CM**		-	+
146.	**CM**		-	+
147.	**CM**		-	+
148.	**CM**		-	+
149.	**CM**		-	+
150.	**CM**		-	+

Faria R. *Evaluation of bacterial leakage along the implant-abutment interface* [doctorate thesis]. São José dos Campos: School of São José dos Campos. UNESP – São Paulo State University; 2008.

ABSTRACT

The aim of this study was to evaluate, in vitro, the bacterial leakage between implant and abutment comparing three kinds of implant-abutments connections: extern hexagon (EH), indexed intern hexagon (IIH) and morse-taper (MT). Under sterile controlled conditions, the tip of the abutment screw was inoculated with *Escherichia coli* culture and then the abutment was placed in position and tightened (20N/cm). The specimen was discarded if an external contamination of the outer surface was observed. Each specimen was incubated in a glass tube containing 2mL of sterile TSB medium at $37^{\circ}C$. The growth of *E. Coli* in the medium was registered every 24h. Once the sample showed cloudy broth, it was individually plated on TSA plates and incubated in an anaerobic chamber at $37^{\circ}C$ for 24h, in order to observe the bacterial growth. Gram test was performed both in the medium and in the culture to certify the presence of *E. Coli* (Gram negative). After 7 days, each test specimen was sampled using a sterile paper point which was incubated in TSA plates and incubated in anaerobic chamber at $37^{\circ}C$ for 24h, to verify bacterial viability. Samples that did not show bacterial viability in the end of the study were eliminated from the final results. After that, there were 38 EH samples, 40 IIH samples and 41 CM samples. The results, in %, of bacterial leakage, were statistically evaluated by multiple comparisons for proportion. The survival curves were analyzed by Kaplan-Meyer method and compared by statistical test of Log-Rank. There was no statistical difference among EH (10,53%), IIH (4,88%) e MT (7,50%). The three survival curves did not differ (p>0.005). It was conclude that the bacterial leakage occurred in a similar way for the three kinds of implant-abutment interface, no matter the assembly configuration.

Keywords: dental implants; prostheses and implants; microbiology; biomechanics.

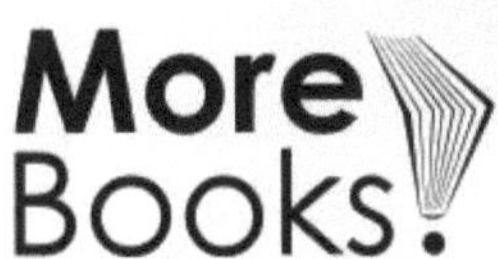

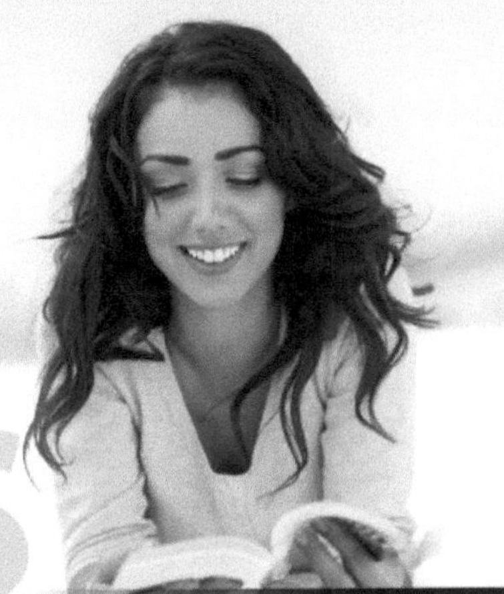

yes
I want morebooks!

Buy your books fast and straightforward online - at one of world's fastest growing online book stores! Environmentally sound due to Print-on-Demand technologies.

Buy your books online at
www.morebooks.shop

Kaufen Sie Ihre Bücher schnell und unkompliziert online – auf einer der am schnellsten wachsenden Buchhandelsplattformen weltweit! Dank Print-On-Demand umwelt- und ressourcenschonend produzi ert.

Bücher schneller online kaufen
www.morebooks.shop

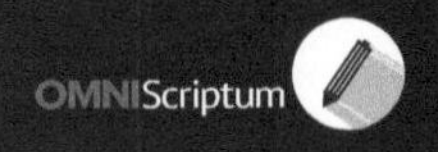